Psychedelic Me
at the
End of Life

"Miller writes personally, emotionally, wisely—unafraid to talk about dark and difficult parts of his own life and enthusiastic about every day remaining. Thoroughly grounded in his own close-to-death experiences and insights gained from his and others' psychedelic journeys, his refreshing understanding of what dying brings to living is healthy and sane. He has given us a needed alternative to our current death-phobic and death-denying usual narrative. He makes a strong case for benefitting from different psychedelic plants and fungi, most of which can reconnect people to the underlying unity in which some parts are being born and some dying but none are ever lost. This is a deeply uplifting, clear, and compassionate guide to dying and how psychedelics, used correctly, diminish our fears about approaching the door that opens at the end of our life."

JAMES FADIMAN, PH.D., MICRODOSE RESEARCHER
AND AUTHOR OF *THE PSYCHEDELIC EXPLORER'S GUIDE*

"A masterful overview of an area of vital importance to our modern world rapidly attracting interest and support. Through his own moving life stories and those of his friends, colleagues, and patients, Miller shares insights on how we may more effectively approach and prepare for the end of life. He wisely states that psychedelics under optimal conditions have a unique application for those mired in psychospiritual suffering and asserts that these are existential medicines of inestimable value. This book is a valuable resource and contribution to the growing field of psychedelic medicine along with our ever-present struggle to find meaning and value to our lives while we still inhabit this mortal coil."

CHARLES S. GROB, M.D., PROFESSOR OF PSYCHIATRY
AT UCLA SCHOOL OF MEDICINE

"From my earliest exposure to psychedelics, I have always carried the pivotal understanding that they showed to me: that death has a bad reputation but is perfectly safe. In *Psychedelic Medicine at the End of Life*, Miller has supported and elaborated upon that perspective, integrating his clinical expertise, his personal experiences, his appreciation for the developing body of research, and his encounters with a unified vision of reality in a book that will be instructive and inspiring to readers from a wide variety of backgrounds and disciplines."

MARIAVITTORIA MANGINI, PH.D., FNP, NURSE, AUTHOR, AND
INVESTIGATOR OF PSYCHEDELIC-ASSISTED THERAPIES

"Miller starts with a gripping and inspiring story and then continues to ply us with vital information. Psychedelics may offer a mini-death rehearsal, offering a glimpse of spiritual oneness, enabling us to be less afraid at the end of our lives. This peacefulness resonates with family and friends, allowing us to stay connected to loved ones throughout the process."

JULIE HOLLAND, M.D., PSYCHIATRIST, EDITOR OF
THE POT BOOK, AND AUTHOR OF *GOOD CHEMISTRY*

"This inspiring book is semi-autobiographical as Miller shares several personal brushes with death and his experiences with psychedelic substances such as morning glory seeds, LSD, DMT, and MDMA. He includes episodes and insights from his academic career and from his work as a clinical psychologist. As he relates his life story, Miller weaves in commentary from interviews with experts in psychedelic research. A captivating read for those interested in this field."

NICHOLAS V. COZZI, PH.D., SCIENTIST AND EDUCATOR

"We needed a guidebook on how to face the end of our lives with the wise application of psychedelic medicine. Dr. Richard Louis Miller is the people's psychologist. His kind voice, six decades of requisite personal and professional experience, and relentless dedication to the very best for all shines through in this book. May reading it help you and your loved ones on your journey toward transcendence."

SUNIL K. AGGARWAL, M.D., PH.D., FAAPMR, FAAHPM,
CODIRECTOR OF AIMS INSTITUTE

Psychedelic Medicine at the End of Life

Dying without Fear

Dr. Richard Louis Miller

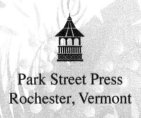

Park Street Press
Rochester, Vermont

Park Street Press
One Park Street
Rochester, Vermont 05767
www.ParkStPress.com

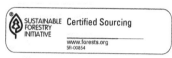

Text stock is SFI certified

Park Street Press is a division of Inner Traditions International

Cataloging-in-Publication Data for this title is available from the Library of Congress

ISBN 978-1-64411-981-5 (print)
ISBN 978-1-64411-982-2 (ebook)

Printed and bound in the United States by Lake Book Manufacturing, LLC
The text stock is SFI certified. The Sustainable Forestry Initiative® program promotes sustainable forest management.

10 9 8 7 6 5 4 3 2 1

Text design and layout by Kenleigh Manseau
This book was typeset in Garamond Premier Pro with Kepler Std and Neuzeit Grotesk used as display typefaces

To send correspondence to the author of this book, mail a first-class letter to the author c/o Inner Traditions • Bear & Company, One Park Street, Rochester, VT 05767, and we will forward the communication.

Scan the QR code and save 25% at InnerTraditions.com. Browse over 2,000 titles on spirituality, the occult, ancient mysteries, new science, holistic health, and natural medicine.

Contents

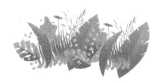

PART ONE
THE CASE FOR PSYCHEDELICS
AT THE END OF LIFE

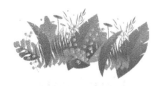

PART TWO

THE STEPS TO DYING GRACEFULLY

Foreword

Rick Doblin, Ph.D.

In 1972, the same year my friend and colleague Dr. Richard Louis Miller was founding The Health Sanctuary at Wilbur Hot Springs, I was an eighteen-year-old college freshman having my first transformative experiences with LSD and mescaline. While difficult to put into words, those journeys opened my eyes to a profound underlying interconnectedness—the revelation that our individual consciousness is merely part of something far vaster and more primordial.

Dr. Miller's book *Psychedelic Medicine at the End of Life* arrives at a pivotal moment to explore how we can apply these powerful medicines to one of the most universal of human experiences: death. Through six decades of practice and personal insights, his work emphasizes the importance of open discussions around dying as a means to reduce suffering. Richard questions the cultural forces that have created the fear of death and advocates for the acceptance of death as being another part of the life cycle.

This perspective resonates with what I've witnessed—that creating conscious spaces for preparation can change the way we relate to mortality.

My teenage psychedelic experiences revealed what I immediately recognized as potential antidotes to society's most pernicious ills: tribalism, prejudice, and fundamentalism. The boundaries of identity and ideology seemed to dissolve in the presence of that indivisible essence we all emanate from. I intuited that a wider embrace of such unitive perspectives could catalyze profound shifts in how we relate to ourselves, each other, and our precious planet.

In the decades since I've seen firsthand how psychedelics can facilitate profound psychological shifts and openings. One of the most memorable instances was in 1984, facilitating an MDMA session for a close friend whose partner was dying of cancer. At the time, he lay consumed by opiate fog, unable to muster the clarity for a final meaningful connection.

The MDMA synergized with the painkillers in an unexpected way—rather than exacerbating the stupor, it elevated his cognition into a shockingly lucid state. With profound presence, he was able to share parting words and emotional closures with his partner. He passed away just three days later, but for the surviving partner, that experience remained one of the most precious and fundamentally important they had shared.

It struck me then that if psychedelics could offer such poignant grace to the dying, this capstone of life may actually be one of their most sacred domains of healing potential. Too often, our culture's aversion to mortality creates bitterness at the end of life, robbing the dying and their families of richly appreciating the journey, making amends, achieving closure, and preparing for their final rites of passage with open-hearted acceptance.

I do not raise such possibilities merely as hypothetical philosophizing. Clinical research from institutions working to bring psychedelics through modern scientific and medical channels, like the non-profit I founded in 1986 and of which I am currently president, the Multidisciplinary Association for Psychedelic Studies (MAPS), has demonstrated the remarkable efficacy of psychedelic medicines in treating forms of distress, such as post-traumatic stress disorder, which many individuals in the process of dying often suffer from.

MAPS's Phase 3 trials found that MDMA-assisted therapy helped two-thirds of participants with severe PTSD no longer qualify for a diagnosis of PTSD and develop a more open, appreciative relationship to life itself.

Psilocybin and LSD have shown similarly stunning results in research trials treating anxiety and depression in terminal cancer patients. Novel imaging studies have revealed these kinds of non-ordinary states of consciousness arise from a precise neurological mechanism: the deactivation of the brain's "default mode network"—the neural circuitry that constructs our sense of being a separate narrative self, distinct from others and our environment.

Such findings have catalyzed rapidly expanding scientific interest in psychedelics' capacity to intervene in humans' deep-rooted patterns of existential avoidance, death anxiety, and self-alienation. It seems our consciousness may be more fundamentally laced with these unitive potentials than previously recognized, with psychedelics serving as unique keys for unlocking such expansive domains of experience on a reliable basis.

Of course, navigating these waters requires consummate care and ethical integrity. These are not merely new therapies to be casually prescribed like medications on a doctor's pad. We must construct integrated therapeutic containers spanning preparation, the actual journey, and long-term integration support. This involves fostering environments imbued with trust, safety, and wisdom to help people metabolize the insights that can emerge. *Psychedelic Medicine at the End of Life* provides us with specific details of what is known—and not known—about the use of psychedelic medicines during this transitioning stage of life.

Another vital dimension is how we foster community contexts where the revelations and insights gained through these inner voyages can be thoughtfully unpacked, distilled through poetry and art, woven into the lived fabric of daily experience. Our ability to realize psychedelics' transformative potential for our whole human journey, including death, depends on cultivating these spaces for deep emotional integration. Dr. Miller's work points the way toward building such containers with wisdom and care.

No human process is more ripe for such tenderness and conscious holding than the final transitions we all must one day make. Throughout history, the great spiritual and wisdom traditions have recognized the profound importance of the dying process and have developed intricate rituals, practices, and art forms to facilitate the passage from life to death. Now, practices involving legal psychedelic therapies are emerging to provide a modern perspective on this ages-old human process—supplementing the wisdom of ancient traditions with insights from clinical research on establishing optimal therapeutic containers.

If we can integrate these powerful tools into our mainstream medical system in a holistic manner—as complements to palliative care, pain management, family counseling, and existential processing—I believe we have an extraordinary opportunity before us. Rather than defaulting to needless existential and emotional anguish at the end of life, whole new vistas could open in how we relate to mortality as individuals, families, and a culture. By thoughtfully preparing and skillfully tending the soil of consciousness itself, we can steward our final rites of passage as not merely endpoints but as graceful awakenings into other fields of perspective that affirm our ultimate continuity beyond the physical forms we've temporarily assumed.

Our oldest stories and spiritual maps have long hinted at the healing revelations that can flower through consciousness expansion. Now, we can realize this potential in a way that can transform our relationship to the great journey we're all undertaking. Dr. Miller's *Psychedelic Medicine at the End of Life* is a timely and important contribution to this unfolding renaissance, offering guidance on how we can bring heart, ethics, and skillful care to the final stage of human existence.

RICK DOBLIN, PH.D., is the president of the Multidisciplinary Association for Psychedelic Studies (MAPS), a nonprofit founded in 1986 with the aim of developing legal contexts for the beneficial uses of psychedelics as prescription medicines. His own personal goal is to eventually become a legally licensed psychedelic therapist.

Prologue

Disgraced president Richard Nixon declared what he called the War on Drugs in 1972. This so-called war was a despicable subterfuge. As John Erlichman, Nixon's closest advisor, told Harper's Magazine reporter Dan Baum years later in 2016:

> We knew we couldn't make it illegal to be either against the war or black, but by getting the public to associate the hippies with marijuana and blacks with heroin, and then criminalizing both heavily, we could disrupt those communities. We could arrest their leaders, raid their homes, break up their meetings, and vilify them night after night on the evening news. Did we know we were lying about the drugs? Of course we did.

There never was a War on Drugs. In reality, there was a war on people of color and people called hippies. Both groups, their families and us all, have suffered mightily from this War on People. What do you think of such a president? Our criminal president, Richard Nixon, was a high-alert warning to us all regarding the type of person we elect to our highest office. History, from Julius Caesar onward, reveals how rapidly and easily a republic can become a dictatorship. For decades, Nixon's War on Drugs made it nearly impossible to do scientific research on psychedelic medicines. Miles of red tape and harsh criminal penalties scared most scientists away from their scientific study.

However, even within this totalitarian atmosphere, there were still a small number of rigorously designed studies on psychedelic medicines allowed, conducted by gentle yet persistent and career-courageous scientists almost all of whom are featured in this book and my 2017 book, *Psychedelic Medicine: The Healing Powers of LSD, MDMA, Psilocybin, and Ayahuasca*. I am pleased that psychedelic science has progressed enough to be able to share what this present book is about, psychedelic medicine at the end of life.

We have enough definitive evidence of both the psychophysical and spiritual benefits of certain psychedelic substances to warrant their classification as medicines. Psychedelic science, and those of us advocating for the science, have come a long way but the road ahead is even longer. It feels quite odd for me to be saying these words here in the United States, which I grew up believing was a beacon of liberty for our planet, only to find that we are no different from any country where political corruption rules over science.

Take heed: just because we are experiencing what is optimistically being called a scientific renaissance or even a psychedelic renaissance does not mean that we are free to breathe the air of liberty. Let us always be mindful that even marijuana, which has no reliable evidence of causing fatal overdoses, remains illegal at the federal level—with over 300,000 arrests for possession in 2020—while cigarettes, responsible for 480,000 deaths, and alcohol, with 140,000 deaths, are legal. Does that seem rational to you? It certainly does not seem rational to me. And if our laws are not based on rationality and science, what are they based on? Are we living at the whim of those who make their careers getting elected to office? And, if so, do we want to continue living this way? Sure, those of us who are white can skate by under racist corruption, but for how long do we wish to skate when the very air we all share and breathe is being stifled by small-minded professional politicians who make their living running for office as politicians? If you are a person of color, do you want to continue to be profiled every time you leave your home?

Our clear lesson is that if and when we ever again elect a Nixon type to high office in our government, we could quickly see a roll back of many humanitarian laws along with scientific research. Hell fire and brimstone are only an election away.

This book serves as a reference for those considering the use of psychedelic medicines and also as a strong caution light to all Americans. When a criminal, such as a Nixon, was able to fool "we the people" into electing him president, untold lives were destroyed, scientists were blocked from conducting experiments on the potential medicinal benefits of certain plants, fungi, and laboratory chemicals, and the public was denied access to medicines demonstrated to be superior to what continues to be available. This last matter is perhaps the most critical. Millions of Americans, and people around the world, have been denied access to psychedelic medicines already proven to be beneficial and well within established safety zones.

One of our most important tasks as citizens is to be ever mindful of those we elect to lead us.

In the words most often attributed to the great American hero Thomas Jefferson, "eternal vigilance is the price of liberty."

PART ONE

THE CASE FOR PSYCHEDELICS AT THE END OF LIFE

CHAPTER 1

Ego Death

A BRUSH WITH DEATH ON THE HIGHWAY

"Stay with me. Call me a helicopter. I'm going to live."

Lying on cold, black pavement, I slowly opened my eyes.

What had begun as another ordinary Sunday morning motorcycle ride turned into a race against the clock to get from my remote location near Bodega Bay on California's North Coast to the nearest hospital in Santa Rosa, California—some 30 miles away.

Just moments prior, I had rounded a curve on the winding roads of Highway 1 and was hit head-on by a large Winnebago recreational vehicle that had drifted into my lane. The Winnebago ran completely over my legs, crushing them both. Then, in the span of a few minutes, I made peace with my imminent demise only to be offered a renewed life, which I gratefully accepted.

My first recollection after the impact was lying on the highway with my eyes shut, watching a bright blinking red light on my inner screen. Alarm bells filled my consciousness.

I tried to lift my left leg and my left foot came up and hit me in the face. The lower half of my leg, below the knee, seemed completely severed from the upper half. The same was true of my right leg.

I became aware of being in large shock and, also, of the necessity to stabilize myself if I were to live.

Immediately, I began doing well-practiced diaphragmatic breathing exercises to achieve some homeostasis and thereby prevent myself from going further into shock and losing consciousness. I knew that regulating my oxygen supply was crucial. Stretched out on my back, with my eyes closed, I was breathing and watching the pulsating red lights in my consciousness as they seemed to get stronger and more urgent.

While breathing slowly and steadily from my abdomen, I flashed back to my training at the Esalen Institute in the 1960s—some twenty years prior—where I had learned, from Bernie Gunther, Gia Fu Feng, Charlotte Selver, and Charles Brooks to regulate my breath and thereby self-regulate my emotions. Over the years, I practiced breath control regularly, absorbing the breathing technique into my being, to regulate my emotions and bring my body's involuntary responses under my conscious control. This time, I was using diaphragmatic breath control to stave off an involuntary stress response that threatened to take my life. Hyperventilation—a normal response to severe bodily trauma—would have further destabilized me and put me into deeper shock, at which point I likely would have lost conscious control over my breathing and everything else.

As I lay there breathing, I could see myself drifting away—out of my body and into the universe.

I assumed this was the end and made my peace with that possibility. Having made peace with what we call death during my first LSD experience in 1965, I was neither fearful nor anxious; I let myself go. And as I relaxed, I once again saw myself drifting off into the darkness of the universe.

I thought, "Okay, this is it. I'm saying goodbye."

As I left my body, the pain from my crushed legs vanished completely. I had the sensation of existing without a physical body. There was no light at the end of the tunnel. It was just big and black and dark—like a dreamless sleep.

Next, I had a vision of myself sitting, strapped into a wheelchair, with a blanket over my legs, meeting with a patient in my office.

A deep voice rang out from within the universe and said to me, "You can still make a contribution."

When I heard this voice, everything changed. I felt a tear well up in my eye, I could still make a contribution. I still had value. I reversed course and watched myself come back from the great darkness; back from the abyss, back to the cold hard pavement and the waves of pain.

All around me, my fellow motorcycle riders were screaming.

Like a scene from the movies, they just kept yelling: "Open your eyes! Open your eyes!"

So, I opened my eyes and asked them to call a helicopter.

"I am going to make it," I said.

THE FIRST EGO DEATH (MICHIGAN, 1965)

In this book, I will share my personal experiences, over a period of fifty-nine years, as well as the latest research demonstrating how psychedelics can transform people's relationship with death by helping them overcome, anxiety, fear, and depression and embrace life more fully.

There is an inscription I resonate with above the door of St. Paul's Monastery on Mount Athos in Macedonia, Northern Greece, dating back to the tenth century. It reads:

"If you die before you die, you won't die when you die."

Several decades before I was run over by the Winnebago, an early experience with psychedelics had given me the first preview of death—a dress rehearsal if you will—that prepared me for my many subsequent brushes with death.

There was that time when I nearly flew off a cliff. I was trailing two young motorcycle riders on my BMW R1000 Paris-Dakar motorcycle on our way to a BMW motorcycling gathering. As I came around a steep curve, I hit a patch of loose rocks and lost control of the motorcycle. I high-sided, flew forward over the bike, and headed toward the edge of the cliff. I saw the face of an old bearded man in front of me, and I heard a loud roaring growl come out of me from very deep inside.

I landed on the edge of the cliff with my upper body hanging over the abyss and my heavy legs holding me on the ground. The bike was next to me, one wheel over the edge. I got up, picked up the bike, and continued the ride with a broken collarbone.

However, the experience that stands out the most of all my encounters with death was my very first one while under the influence of LSD (Lysergic Acid Diethylamide). At no point in this psychedelic experience was I at risk of actually dying, and yet it came closest to giving me the actual experience of my own death. Ego death is not to be confused with physical death, but we can learn a great deal about the latter from the former.

At the time, in the second half of the 1960s, teaching life at the University of Michigan in Ann Arbor was like a scene out of the TV show *Ozzie and Harriet*. All the faculty seemed to want a pink princess telephone, a white picket fence, and two cars in the garage. The locals believed that if you worked for either Ford or General Motors you were a happy camper. Campus life then was all about going to football games after lining up early in the morning to get a good seat and drinking beer at the local tavern.

It was before the Summer of Love and well before Nixon and the so-called War on Drugs. From my happy life in middle America, I knew little about what was going on in Haight-Ashbury in 1966, and I don't think many others did either. I had short hair and my work uniform was what I thought was proper clothing—a three-piece tweed suit made of herringbone material. The counterculture or hippie movement had not arrived yet, except in glimpses.

Due to the close relationship between the psychology departments at the University of Michigan and Harvard, I became aware of the psychedelic science research that had been conducted by Timothy Leary and Richard Alpert before they were fired from Harvard University in 1963. I obtained Leary's famous revision of the Tibetan Book of the Dead, which inspired me to conduct my own experiment in the centuries-old tradition of scientists using themselves as subjects in experiments. In the back of Leary and Alpert's book was a reference to a method for extracting psychoactive substances from heavenly blue or pearly gates morning glory seeds.

In accord with Leary's prescription, along with a close, older friend, Alan Pinsince, I ingested four hundred LSA-laden heavenly blue morning glory seeds (Convolvulaceae containing certain fungi in the genus

Periglandula). Just getting such a large number of morning glory seeds down my throat was itself quite challenging and something I hardly recommend. Swallowing the four hundred seeds was just the beginning. This experience changed the course of my life.

At one point during the experience when I felt scared, the thought crossed my mind, "What if there was some kind of adulterant in what I took?"

I didn't get the seeds from a laboratory.

About an hour into the experience, I began thinking to myself, "I'm really dying."

The scariest part was feeling like I was going to die as soon as I let go. However, some voice of wisdom in me said, "If you are going to die, you are going to die and there is nothing you can do. Just let go and let it happen."

So I let go and let "it" happen for the first time. I have done "it" more than once, and each time I do, I always try to let go and let "it" happen again.

What is this mysterious "it" that many have called ego death?

After letting go, I found myself in a state of consciousness without a body. Although I was still aware, I felt unified with everything in the universe. I was having a transcendent experience.

I had no sense of my physical body, and my eyes were closed the whole time—much like the years-later near-death experience lying on the highway after the motorcycle accident. I had no awareness of the room or anything material around me. It was as if I were an electromagnetic light being.

Ever since, I have identified with Alex Grey's paintings depicting us as electrified beings. That experience of what is called ego death changed my view of death and life.

Once I felt like I experienced consciousness as separate from my body, I became open to the possibility that when I actually physically die, I may still have some form of consciousness.

During that journey I went back in time. I observed small groups of people around the world growing and evolving, from the caves and into villages, then towns, and then rapidly becoming cities. I watched these cities become feudal areas, and eventually kingdoms and countries. It was like watching a film on rapid time-lapse showing the progress and the development of culture. I saw countries aligning with other countries and becoming larger political unions until the entire world was unified.

I had a sense of an all-encompassing feeling of interconnectedness with every other human being and everything on the planet. It changed me from seeing us as living on the planet, to seeing us as being a part of the planet. Our planet was no longer a ball that we're sitting on but rather an organism that we're part of and incorporated into.

Prior to this experience, I had believed that death was like falling asleep without dreaming. However, I became fully aware that death may not be the end and it is something to accept rather than to fear. From this initial experience it was easy to see that, as therapists, we could provide people with similar experiences prior to death to help them acclimate and accept that death is part of our developmental process and nothing to fear.

My first psychedelic experience served as a monumental educator. Since then, through my continued psychedelic experiments and ego deaths, I have learned to follow the legendary psychedelic scientist Bill Richards's advice and when the situation calls for it, I let myself die.

WHEN THE DOCTOR KNOCKS

Flash forward fifty years from that first psychedelic experience and I found myself once again confronted with my own mortality. A few months after my eighty-second birthday I was sitting in my doctor's office, feeling healthy and upbeat. Despite the vibrant health I felt, the doctor's visit was a stark reminder that understanding one's physical well-being requires more than just positive feelings; it needs a deep dive into the empirical world of medical data.

I enjoy collecting all kinds of physiological information about myself because I like learning through data. I regularly inform myself of my inner workings via hematology tests, lipid tests, and other measurements such as blood pressure, heart rate, blood oxygen, body temperature, ECG (electrocardiogram), and eGFR (estimated Glomerular Filtration Rate).

During a routine heart examination I was informed that I was in heart failure. My left ventricle was failing to pump enough oxygenated blood to my system to sustain it. The percentage of blood pumped from the left ventricle, with each stroke, is called the ejection fraction. The normal range of ejection fraction is 55–70 percent. My ejection fraction was 34 percent. I researched heart failure and the severity of my condition, and discovered that this was life threatening. I realized that at any moment, my heart might stop providing the oxygen required for sustaining life and I would cease.

Just before this routine cardiology appointment, I had pressed my dermatologist about a persistent spot on my right temple. For over a year, he had told me it was just a basal cell, and to remove it, he was spraying it with liquid nitrogen. I wasn't sure his diagnosis was accurate.

I finally said, "The spot is not going away. Maybe we should send it in for a biopsy."

While I waited for the results of the biopsy, I received the heart failure diagnosis.

Then the biopsy results came back: nodular malignant melanoma.

The next day, while giving blood at the hospital for further testing, when a nurse trainee glanced down at my chart, I saw the blood drain from her face.

I looked at her and said, "What just happened? You look like you're in shock."

She hesitatingly said, "Well, I saw your diagnosis. My aunt got that same diagnosis six weeks ago, and she died yesterday."

I went home and, together with my wife, googled the specific cancer. Sure enough, the nodular form of metastatic melanoma is capable of killing in six weeks. And because of the misdiagnosis, I'd already had this melanoma for an entire year.

So there I was, dealing with two life-threatening diagnoses. I suspect that many people in my situation would have received this news like a gut punch. Understandably so, but not me.

I had conquered the fear of death with my early self-experiments.

By the time I received these two life threatening diagnoses, I had already come to believe that we make too big of a deal about death as it is simply just another part of the natural developmental process. We are born, we live, and then we die. We don't know where we came from and we don't know what, if anything, is next. This outlook dawned on me during my first experience with the morning glory seeds in 1965. Afterward, I saw the possibility that our essence transcends the physical form. My perspective shifted profoundly—no longer did I view the body's demise as definitely the end. While devastating emotionally for loved ones, death now seemed to possibly be a transition between modes of being, the nature of which remains a mystery to the living.

Viewing death as just one turn in life's cycle fortified me immeasurably when facing my own diagnoses. Though potentiality shocking, I received the news with equanimity, thanks to the wisdom gleaned from my previous ego death experiences. By confronting mortality head-on early and often through psychedelics, I was prepared to embrace life undeterred by its impermanence.

I've often asked myself throughout my life, "How much time of my life do I want to spend dealing with my death?"

My answer is: Very little. I want to live my life and then experience my death.

I have come to speculate that the fundamental basis of all fears is the fear of death. I believe fear is bad for both physical and mental health so I've done everything I can to face my fears, expose myself to them, and avoid living fearfully.

Toward this end, I've found psychedelic medicines to be an irreplaceable tool for searching out fear within myself, confronting it, feeling it, expressing it, and evaporating it.

Whenever I embark on a search mission to find and confront my fears, I inevitably come back to the fear of death. I am constantly looking for any lurking fears that may affect me, and as I drill down, there is always the fear of death at the bottom.

Have I permanently eliminated every iota of fear in my psyche around death? No. But by age fifty, when the Winnebago ran over me and crushed my legs, I'd had plenty of practice confronting my fear of dying.

After the motorcycle accident, I dealt with the fear and post-traumatic stress of getting hurt again in a crash. Despite the accident's severity, I was determined to not succumb to a generalized gradient of fear. I was concerned that the trauma could cause long-term Post-Traumatic Stress Disorder (PTSD). Would I be able to drive on a freeway again without triggering a fear response? Would I ride a motorcycle again?

After getting out of the wheelchair—which the doctors told me I'd be confined to for life—and learning to walk again, one of the things I did was strap my crutches onto a motorcycle and return to the exact place where the accident happened. I practiced making that same turn over and over, perfectly, until the trauma of crashing faded. I felt it was important to heal the trauma and replace it with a perfect turn. One could use this as a life slogan: heal the trauma and replace it with a perfect turn.

When I received the dual life-threatening diagnoses of heart failure and metastatic melanoma I stayed in the present moment in which everything in my system was functioning. I continued my daily routine of exercising, eating, reading, making love, hosting my internet radio broadcast, *Mind Body Health & Politics*, writing books, and consulting with patients.

My mantra was this: So long as I am able to function, I'm going to go on with my daily life as it is.

If anything, the experience motivated me to seize each day with even more vigor. Determined to live, I also created a special program to attempt to fix my failing heart.

I credit much of my positive attitude to my rich history of personal experimentation with psychedelics. Some say that these mind-altering substances are merely a crutch, or offer an illusory solution—leading to a sort of blissed-out resignation to our ultimate fate. This stereotype is—in my experience—mistaken. Psychedelics have been the catalysts to squeeze as much living out of life as possible. I have taken each occasion of a near-death experience to double down on this gift we're given. After all—as far as I know—we only get one time around, so it is in our interest to get the most out of life as possible.

SEIZING THE DAYS

All my brushes with death have had something in common. I have come out on the other side, often against the odds. Chance may have played a role, but it's not the full story.

Many people believe that using psychedelics for end of life is about complacency or resignation in the face of something we should rightly fear. However, my experience has been the opposite. Confronting the inevitability of death through psychedelics has motivated me to live more fully and seize each day as a gift.

Immediately after the major motorcycle accident, I saw that I was being given a choice between living and making a contribution or letting the curtain close after fifty years of full and grateful living. I chose to write a second act, beginning with the decision to regulate my breathing and opening my eyes.

The next decision was to collect myself enough to have the onlookers ride as fast as they could to find a telephone and call for a helicopter (there were no cell phones back then). Then I closed my eyes again, telling those around me that I had work to do—the inner work of regulating my breathing and my internal state.

Upon the helicopter's arrival at the hospital, I was immediately taken to the emergency room where they cut off my clothing. As I lay naked on the table, someone yanked on my left leg.

"EYAAA!" I screamed. "What was that?"

A man came to me and said, "Hi, I'm Dr. Bodner and I just tried to realign your left leg, which was completely dislocated."

I said, "Well, I think it would have been more cordial if you had introduced yourself before you yanked on my leg?"

And he said, "Well, we are going to have to amputate your legs."

"Really?" I asked.

"Yes," he said. "Do you know what happened to you?"

I said, "Of course. I kept myself conscious the whole time. I thought I had to keep myself from going further into shock and dying."

He said, "Well, you did a good job, but we're still going to have to amputate your legs."

I asked, "Why?"

He explained, "Because you were run over by a Winnebago. You could be bleeding out."

I replied, "Doctor, from the time I was run over to the time the helicopter arrived and transported me here, and by the time you arrived, if I was going to bleed out, I would have already. How is it possible that I can speak with you? We need an angiogram to determine what's going on in my legs."

He said, "Okay, I'll do that, but you won't be able to control your legs."

I asked, "Well, how come I can do *this*?"

I showed him how I could wiggle my toes.

After they performed the angiogram, he returned with a bewildered look and said, "I can't explain it, but the circulatory system in your legs is intact."

I said, "I guess we have some carpentry to do."

The first of several surgeries lasted fifteen and a half hours. I awoke in intensive care and was told my legs were saved but that I would be wheelchair-bound for life.

I responded by saying, "I will finish a triathlon within two years."

As soon as I got out of intensive care and was able, I began driving the wheelchair around the hospital to maintain my upper-body strength as my legs atrophied. After three weeks in the hospital, I returned home and immediately began seeing patients again. I knew that making a contribution was critical for my recovery.

To rehabilitate myself, I went for long rides in the wheelchair and used dynamic tension to maintain strength in my legs. After six months in the wheelchair, I took my first step and cried sweet tears, for I knew that if I could take one step, I could learn to walk again. A few months later I was out of the wheelchair and walking. Then, I was able to drive to the gym and resume weight training. And yes, I completed two triathlons within two years of the crash. For the running event, I used special T-Bar crutches.

Using the same crutches, creating a quadrapod, I later completed San Francisco's 7.5-mile bridge-to-bridge race (Bay Bridge to Golden Gate), finishing 2,997th in a field of 3,000 bipodal entrants.

Thirty-two years later, rather than accepting my two grim diagnoses as reasons to resign myself to the looming prospect of death, I once again kicked into high gear, calmly and deliberately doing everything I could to improve my prospects for survival. Psychedelic insights supported peace of mind rather than panic or distress, allowing me to focus my energy on constructive actions to improve my prognosis. I doubled down on healthy lifestyle factors, cheerfully underwent multiple educational surgeries, and pursued novel treatments with optimism. My equanimity was built upon a foundation of psychedelic experiences showing me that consciousness exists beyond the body. As terrifying as physical death might seem, I've learned to avoid over-identifying with my mortal frame.

Instead of following professional advice to cut back on my aerobic exercise program due to my failing heart, I doubled my aerobic exercise and worked out on the elliptical machine for sixty minutes, seven days a week. I had already been more than 90 percent vegan and further reduced my intake of non-vegan foods. I decreased my very light alcohol consumption to almost zero and drank half my body weight in ounces of water daily. Furthermore, I worked on improving my mental state and took the following medications:

Entresto 5mg, twice daily
Carvedilol 3.125mg, twice daily,
Apixiban 20mg, twice daily
Crestor 20 mg, daily
LSD 12ug, twice weekly and 100µg, twice monthly

Six months later, I took an echocardiogram, and my ejection fraction was 55 percent—in the low-normal range. Six months after that, it was still low to normal at 55 percent. Another six months later, my ejection fraction was 63 percent, placing me in the seventy-second percentile. My cardiologist, Dr. Anan Soni, told me I had a normal heart.

With regard to the threat of the nodular malignant melanoma: After the cancer was removed from my face, I underwent a surgical procedure called sentinel lymphadenectomy. In this procedure, radioactive material is injected into the melanoma area, followed by a biopsy of the nearest lymph gland. This method determines whether the cancer has migrated to the lymph gland and then most likely metastasized. The biopsy revealed there was no metastasis during the year the cancer had been present. I was cancer free.

I asked my excellent surgeon, Dr. Jonathan George, of the Medical School at the University of San Francisco (UCSF), who performed the surgery and the biopsy, "How did I live a whole year with this rapidly spreading nodular malignant melanoma that can kill in six weeks? How am I still here?"

Dr. George replied, "Your body built a capsule around the melanoma and prevented it from spreading the entire time."

I asked "How certain are you that I am cancer-free?"

He said, "Ninety to ninety-five percent certain."

I asked further, "How can we be one hundred percent certain?"

He suggested, "Take a PET-CT scan."

I took the PET-CT scan, and it was clear.

I presently enjoy a happy, healthy heart, and there is no cancer in my system. While psychedelics didn't directly heal me, the lack of fear or distress related to the diagnoses allowed me to focus fully on lifestyle changes and medical treatment.

EMBRACING TRANSFORMATION

Today, at eighty-five, I am healthy. As predicted in my earlier vision while lying on the freeway after having been crushed by the Winnebago, I have continued making a contribution to the world as a clinical psychologist seeing patients, an internet radio host, an author, and until recently as the owner-operator of the health sanctuary I founded in 1972 at Wilbur Hot Springs in Northern California. I walk on two legs, continue to do aerobics six days a week, and lift weights four days a week. Yet beyond the physical obstacles I've overcome, there is an underlying attitude toward life that stems from a deeper kind of knowing.

In his book *Stranger in a Strange Land*, Robert Heinlein introduced the concept of "grokking," which refers to a type of understanding that goes beyond mere thinking and feeling. Grokking is a profound way of knowing, accessible only through our highest consciousness. Psychedelic substances can facilitate the experience of grokking, thereby creating a transformative effect on our entire being, from our beliefs to our thoughts and emotions.

To illustrate this, let's consider an example. Imagine you had always believed that the world is flat. Then, you travel to the supposed "edge" of the world and realize that there is no edge—that you can keep going around the Earth. This realization, experienced at the deepest level of your being, is undeniable and transformative. It challenges your previous belief about the world and replaces it with a new understanding that the Earth is actually round, not flat. This new understanding can then have a ripple effect on the rest of your beliefs, thoughts, and emotions, changing how you interact with the world and the people around you. You come to realize that you can hold a deep belief about the world, which is mistaken.

Ever since my experience of ego death in 1965, nearly sixty years ago, I have never looked at death the same way. The difference is as stark as perceiving the world as round instead of flat. My ability to confront the real possibility of death with peace came from profound experiences that I hope will, someday, be accessible to anyone who wishes to undergo a similar transformation.

There is a part of me that does not want to talk, think, or write extensively, about death. To dwell on death, while alive, seems a waste of time that could be better spent living. I endeavor to spend every day, if not every moment, living; and when death comes, I will embrace it—live it and die it. I intend to live my death to the fullest. I may even create a pre-death party and then die at a time and place of my choosing.

I am contemplating a transitioning party while I am still alive, rather than an after-the-fact funeral with me not in attendance. Think of it yourself. Imagine attending your own transitioning party, where each family member and friend tells their favorite memory about you and concludes by wishing you a bon voyage. Some might prefer a small private event while others might choose a Zoom farewell gathering. We can each create our own goodbye experience, but I can guarantee you this:

for you, even an average farewell party that you attend will be more ful-filling than the most glorious funeral held while you are underground.

Loving life, even in my most despairing moments, I am doing as much, or more, to stay healthy than ever before. I aspire to live to 111 but recognize that our time on this planet is finite, for none of us can predict how much time we have.

For more than fifty years, the United States government misguid-edly suppressed scientific research on psychedelic medicines. My ini-tial experiences in the 1960s, while profound, remained outside of the realm of accepted research except for those small circles that have main-tained the ancient tradition of scientific self-experimentation. However, the tide of suppression of science is shifting. In recent years, a growing number of scientists have courageously engaged in psychedelic research after decades of taboos. Slowly, yet surely, the world is being granted access to knowledge and understanding of the benefits of psychedelic medicines for a wide variety of conditions, including, but not limited to, PTSD, depression, and anxiety.

These researchers' foundation of rigorous evidence has brought us to the cusp of getting MDMA (3,4-Methylenedioxymethamphetamine, aka "ecstasy") approved for legal medical use possibly before this book is published. Psychedelic plants and fungi have already been decriminal-ized in Colorado and Oregon, as well as in several cities. The work of psychedelic scientists offers new hope for the dying by showing psyche-delics' power to alleviate end-of-life psychological and existential dis-tress. While modern medicine addresses symptom alleviation the actual healing of emotional/spiritual anguish remains within the domain of psychedelics. In this book, I will interweave commentary from my interviews with a wide selection of carefully curated scientists, from many professions, who specialize in psychedelic research. Where a quote is present but does not include a citation, it originates from an interview between the interviewee and myself. To listen to my interviews in full, visit my website at mindbodyhealthpolitics.org. My archives are open source without built-in fees.

Changes in the legal landscape are providing new opportunities for law-abiding citizens to exercise their rights to ingest substances of their choice, so long as they do not harm others. While I regard this as a fundamental right, I acknowledge, with sadness, that many will only seek this option at the end of life and only if it carries zero risk of legal consequences. It deeply saddens me that our government has applied the law to the ingestion of substances. Personally and professionally, I find it intolerable that we have elected leaders with such a narrow mindset, sending citizens to prison for nothing more than ingesting a substance. The fact that the government can legally tell me what I can and cannot eat is an insult to the core of my sovereignty and the sovereignty of us all.

In the next chapter, we will explore the work of the pioneers in psychedelic research who are making steady progress toward getting psychedelics approved for the most urgent uses—including the ever-present fear of death that robs so many of precious lifetime. The prominent figures in psychedelic research illuminate these insights so that everyone can face mortality with open eyes and hearts.

CHAPTER 2

From Taboo to Trials

Pioneers of the Psychedelic Renaissance

There are certain topics that are career killers in academia—taboo subjects that threaten the established order. For Professor Ernest Hilgard, a renowned psychologist at Stanford University in the mid-twentieth century, hypnosis was one such subject.

When I was in graduate school in Michigan, Hilgard visited and gave a lecture on hypnosis.

After the lecture, I asked him, "For most of your career, you were studying rats, and just in recent years, you started researching hypnosis. How did that come about?"

He replied, "It was simple. If I had started with hypnosis right away, I wouldn't have had a career. I waited until I was a full professor, and then, after I was tenured, I was able to pursue my real interests."

This cautionary tale has stayed with me for over half a century. When I first took the Morning Glory seeds containing LSA in 1965, I understood its profound potential—not only for healing and extinguishing my fears around death and dying but also for personal growth and creativity.

However, I also understood that embracing this insight could end my career before it even began. Psychedelics were taboo and for specific reason: they threatened to upend centuries-old assumptions about the mind, the self, and human consciousness. People who think for themselves cannot be easily persuaded about their vote. Collectively, we are *bound* by death. Death grips us with fear, and we grip back at it. It seems that below our fear of death, there is another fear of losing our fear. To some, being free of the fear of death sounds frightening.

So, like Hilgard, I waited.

Instead of pursuing my interest in psychedelics as a researcher, I channeled my energy into political activism. Specifically, I advocated for what I believe to be a basic right—the right to ingest anything I want in the privacy of my own home, so long as I do not harm another person.

As an activist, I supported organizations such as the Multidisciplinary Association for Psychedelic Studies (MAPS), founded by my dear friend Rick Doblin; the Drug Policy Alliance (DPA), founded by my friend Ethan Nadelman; the Marijuana Policy Project (MPP), founded by my friend Rob Kampia; and the National Organization for the Reform of Marijuana Laws (NORML), founded by my good acquaintance Keith Stroup. I raised funds for these organizations and had the privilege of sitting on the National Board of Directors for the Marijuana Policy Project."

For over fifty years, I observed how the United States government stigmatized psychedelics through propaganda, disinformation, fear, and the threat of personal prosecution. I have witnessed lives being ruined by misguided laws. For over fifty years, I waited for the cultural winds to shift and for institutions to open their doors again to legitimate scientific exploration of these extraordinary substances. The present revival of psychedelic research has been a long time coming, and, at last, the dark ages of scientific suppression appear to be possibly ending. I say "possibly" because even marijuana possession is still a federal crime and I doubt I will live to see the legalization of LSD, which is arguably the most beneficial psychedelic substance.

This shift is happening in no small part due to the new approach being taken by psychedelic researchers, prioritizing medical and psychological research to alleviate various physical and mental health conditions.

This new era of psychedelic science is confirming what I, as well as many others, learned over fifty-five years ago: that these novel medicines have the potential to revolutionize our understanding and treatment of the human mind and to facilitate creativity. The experiences I had in the

1960s now have the support of numerous clinical trials and brain scans. There are discoveries to be made and lives to transform.

The future of these substances is bright if we have the courage and wisdom to follow where they lead us. However, we have only just begun to understand the promises and potential perils of psychedelics.

THE FIVE STAGES OF THE PSYCHEDELIC RENAISSANCE

Thomas Roberts is a professor emeritus of educational psychology at Northern Illinois University, a pioneer in psychedelic studies, and the author of the book *Mindapps: Multistate Theory and Tools for Mind Design*. He originated the world's first university-cataloged psychedelic course, Foundations of Psychedelic Studies, which he taught for thirty-two years. I have had the privilege of interviewing Roberts on my program *Mind Body Health & Politics* on multiple occasions, to provide his perspective—a big picture view on the state of the still-emerging field of psychedelic studies.

"The Renaissance is just beginning," he tells me. "And it has a long path ahead of it."

My ultimate goal is to make these medicines available to anyone who wishes to use them—not just for therapy or neuroscience, but to enhance creativity, wisdom, and well-being.

But we have had to proceed with caution. Like Hilgard, psychedelic researchers have had to establish their careers before diving into this taboo. Only once there is scientific consensus on safety, efficacy, and ethical use will psychedelics move fully into the light.

The first stage of mainstream acceptance, according to Roberts, will manifest through psychotherapy and neuroscience. This is where most current research is concentrated, establishing the medical potential of psychedelics to treat conditions like PTSD, anxiety, addiction, and the subject matter of this book: end-of-life anxiety and depression.

As more people discover the power of these psychedelic medicines to occasion mystical experiences, we will enter the second stage: the entheogen stage. *Entheogen* is an alternate term for some psychedelic substances, particularly when they are used to induce the mystical or spiritual experience of "the divine within."

We appear to already be crossing the threshold from stage one to stage two, as evidenced by the blossoming of dozens, if not hundreds, of religious groups and underground churches being established to provide access to the psychedelic experience outside of a clinical setting.*

The third stage of the psychedelic renaissance is what Roberts calls the "ideagen" stage—using psychedelics to generate new ideas and ways of thinking. This stage taps into the creative, intellectual, political, and philosophical potential of these substances.

Roberts's fourth and final stage envisions the incorporation of psychedelics into a broader range of mind-enhancement techniques like meditation, breathwork, and neurofeedback. He refers to these as "mind apps"—tools we can employ to unlock the mind's full capabilities.

However, I believe these four stages need a fifth stage if we are to save ourselves from ourselves.

The reality is that we still live in a world dominated by wars, violence, environmental destruction, and monumental income inequality. We live in a capitalist financial system based on a foundation of winners and losers. This reality is poorly masked by a culture of consumerism, where we attempt to fill the voids in our lives with the purchase of mere junk. In 2023, 62 percent of people in the United States lived paycheck to paycheck (Dickler 2023), while those at the top buy $500 million yachts. This income inequality creates monumental emotional distress, beyond measurement, and the Center for Disease Control (CDC) reports that over 72 percent of Americans suffer from overweight or obesity due to their using food as a coping mechanism and to a bottom-line capitalist mentality which sells them cheap, empty calories made of sugar and corn products. These societal issues are fueling epidemics of diseases and death that require both a restructuring of our financial system and the introduction of new and innovative treatments. The use of

---

*For an overview of these new organizations, I recommend consulting Mike Marinacci's 2023 book, *Psychedelic Cults and Outlaw Churches: LSD, Cannabis, and Spiritual Sacraments in Underground America.*

psychedelics to help people overcome fear and embrace life fully is one such innovation that could help address these issues on multiple fronts. After confronting the inevitability of death, people may be motivated to break free from the treadmill of modern consumerism and strive to make a more a positive contribution to their own well-being and that of society.

Reflecting on these observations, I recently wrote to Roberts and proposed the addition of a fifth stage: psychedelic politics.

In this fifth stage, we take the foundational wisdom we have learned from psychedelics, the realization that people and the planet are one, and use this knowledge to create political and governmental frameworks counteracting the present divisive systems. We can create unification czars, similar to the happiness czars in Bhutan. Political decisions would be made based on the degree of unity they foster. Is this an impossible dream? Perhaps. Yet my idealism fuels my optimism, which is important to maintain as the alternatives to optimism are grim.

Psychedelic medicines may offer more than many have imagined—even those of us at the core of the movement to legalize and decriminalize psychedelics. While we, the advocates of this psychedelic renaissance, have made a good start, we must remember that the renaissance is still in its infancy. Roberts's four-stage progression offers a blueprint of sorts, and those of us who want to see these substances legalized for the full range of possible uses must resist the urge to run ahead of ourselves.

Yet with scientific rigor and caution, we can learn from the Ernest Hilgards of the world by following a careful strategy that begins with the first stage: demonstrating the medicinal and psychotherapeutic benefits of psychedelics within existing legal and regulatory structures.

THIS TIME IT MUST BE DONE SAFELY AND SCIENTIFICALLY: THE PIONEERS OF PSYCHEDELIC RESEARCH

The pioneers of this new wave of psychedelic research have shown tremendous courage.

Roland Griffiths, the founding director of the Johns Hopkins Center for Psychedelic and Consciousness Research, is a pioneering scientist in the field of psychedelic research. He risked his reputation to investigate how psychedelics can help treat depression and psychological distress in patients with a life-threatening cancer diagnosis (Griffiths et al. 2016) as well as addiction (Garcia-Romeu et al. 2019).

Prior to his foray into psychedelics, Griffiths spent over thirty years studying mood-altering drugs of abuse. Like Hilgard, this foundation of "approved" research gave him the credibility and security to begin a new research track in his "second act."

When I first interviewed Griffiths on *Mind Body Health & Politics* in 2012, he had only recently begun studying the classic hallucinogens on which research had been actively suppressed since the 1960s.

My 2017 book *Psychedelic Medicine: The Healing Powers of LSD, MDMA, Psilocybin and Ayahuasca* tells the story of how Griffiths and his team at Johns Hopkins secured approval from the government's Institutional Review Board (IRB). This initial approval was stage one before receiving approval by the Food and Drug Administration (FDA) for his proposed study—a revisitation, in 2006, of Dr. Walter Pahnke's famous "Good Friday Experiment" of the 1960s, in which psilocybin reportedly induced religious-like experiences in seminary students.

Griffiths's study was the first serious research in decades to receive FDA approval to study psilocybin in healthy volunteers. His initial findings demonstrated that these substances could be studied safely under carefully controlled conditions. The research provided compelling evidence that, as measured by pre- and post-testing for depression, subjects who received psilocybin showed less signs of clinical depression one year after ingestion and counseling. This research also informed the world that it appears unnecessary to take antidepressants every day of the year, as we have been told by Big Pharma.

As David E. Nichols, a psychopharmacologist and the world's leading LSD researcher, then at Purdue University, wrote in a publication in the *Journal of Psychopharmacology* in 2006:

The [2006] article by Griffiths et al . . . should make all scientists interested in human psychopharmacology sit up and take notice. It is the first well-designed, placebo-controlled, clinical study in more than four decades to examine the psychological consequences of the effects of the hallucinogenic (psychedelic) agent known as psilocybin. In fact, one would be hard pressed to find a single study of psychedelics from any earlier era that was as well done or as meaningful. Perhaps more importantly, despite the notion by many people that psychedelics are nothing more than troublesome drugs of abuse, the present study convincingly demonstrates that, when used appropriately, these compounds can produce remarkable, possibly beneficial, effects that certainly deserve further study.

In the same year, 2006, Harriet de Wit of the Department of Psychiatry at the University of Chicago echoed Nichols's comments:

People have long sought meaning and significance in their lives through a variety of spiritual practices including prayer, fasting, chanting, solitude, and meditation. Historically, some of these practices have included the use of certain psychoactive plants. A common theme of these experiences, with or without the aid of psychoactive agents, has been to free oneself of the bounds of everyday perception and thought in a search for universal truths and enlightenment. To a large extent, this type of subjective and uniquely human experience has enjoyed little credibility in the mainstream scientific world and, thus, has been given little scientific attention. However, it may be time now to recognize these extraordinary subjective experiences, even if they are, at present, not directly verifiable by objective measures and even if they sometimes involve claims about ultimate realities that lie outside the purview of science.

The significance of Griffiths's work at Johns Hopkins cannot be overstated. The institution's prestige within the medical community gave Griffiths's research immediate credibility and helped open doors at other top institutions like the University of California, Los Angeles

(UCLA), where Dr. Charles Grob began conducting early studies of psilocybin (Grob et al. 2011). Inspired by the initial success at Johns Hopkins, Anthony Bossis, along with Dr. Stephen Ross at the School of Medicine at New York University (NYU), began examining psilocybin for end-of-life distress in patients with life-threatening cancer after seeing the initial successes at Johns Hopkins (Ross et al. 2016).

Griffiths, Grob, Bossis, and Ross, among others, can be regarded as the "godfathers" of the psychedelic research renaissance—pioneering clinicians willing to risk their reputations to revive a promising field of study that had been shuttered for decades.

The meticulous accumulation of rigorous evidence by these researchers laid the groundwork for expanding psychedelic therapy to those most in need—including the dying. Their foundational studies established protocols for safe administration and demonstrated significant improvements in quality of life when paired with psychotherapy.

Griffiths, who continued to conduct research into psychedelics for end-of-life distress, faced his own terminal cancer diagnosis with courage, wisdom, and grace. Despite a prognosis of just months left to live, he discussed his condition not with despair but with profound gratitude for the preciousness of each moment. Having guided many through psychedelic encounters with mortality, he walked the path himself, and his personal experience may offer solace to others in similar situations.

Throughout his decades of research, Griffiths has sought to understand the awe-inspiring mystery of human consciousness. Psychedelics offer glimpses into this unfathomable domain that give many a sense of the sacred. Though a man of science, Griffiths embraces the possibility of realities beyond the reach of conventional measurement tools. His life's work illuminates the deep questions that arise at the boundaries of existence.

Griffiths's research has shown psilocybin's power to occasion experiences of unity and transcendence of the ego that translate into clinically significant benefits. His carefully designed studies provide proof of concept—demonstrating that these long-misunderstood and feared substances can be studied responsibly to alleviate psychological suffering when administered with expert guidance.

At Johns Hopkins and other institutions, Griffiths supported the early days of psychedelic science through its challenging early days, leading to today's psychedelic renaissance. As his health declined, he inspired others to approach death with curiosity and courage, instead of giving in to despair. In doing so, Griffiths set an example for those who would soon face the same journey, fostering hope that his work will bring comfort and meaning to many as they approach life's end.

The path forward is clear: we must follow in the footsteps of these pioneers, advancing this research with robust scientific rigor.

THE RENAISSANCE ACCELERATES: NEW TRIALS, NEW HOPE

At the time of my first interview with Griffiths in 2012, psychedelic research was still taboo. The humble man I interviewed had not yet become the subject of *New York Times* profiles. Netflix had not yet released their 2022 miniseries *How to Change Your Mind,* based on Michael Pollan's best-selling 2018 book of the same name. The conversations laid the groundwork for my book, *Psychedelic Medicine,* and were some of the only overviews of the research taking place in the fledgling field of psychedelic research. How far we have come.

Today, psychedelic studies are expanding on multiple fronts. After decades of darkness, psychedelic research is accelerating into the light.

Grob continues his research at UCLA.

At UCSF, Dr. Brian Anderson and his colleagues are exploring psilocybin for depression and Parkinson's. (See the study details in the Woolley 2021 resource.) Anderson, a lead researcher in UCSF's studies on end-of-life anxiety, told me that he's optimistic about integrating these psychedelic molecules into conventional treatment paradigms.

"As a psychiatrist, I'm curious about what we can offer people seeking help for distress and traumas from their past and challenges in their day-to-day life," he says. "Now I want to see how we can best combine medication and evidence-based talk therapies to support people in a structured yet compassionate way."

Guided by science and compassion, these novel treatments are finding a place within mainstream care.

The FDA approval process is designed to ensure that these powerful medicines meet the highest standards of safety and efficacy before being made available to the public.

> Phase 1 trials establish basic safety and dosage parameters in small groups. Researchers define a dosage range and identify possible side effects. As of 2024, psilocybin and MDMA have now passed Phase 1, demonstrating an acceptable safety profile in controlled settings.
>
> In Phase 2, the goal is to validate the concept by showing efficacy (i.e., tangible benefits) for a specific condition in a small population. Promising Phase 2 trials are now investigating the use of psilocybin for depression, addiction, and Alzheimer's disease.
>
> Phase 3 is the final step before the FDA considers the approval to market a new drug — attempting to demonstrate real-world effectiveness through large, multisite trials.

MAPS is currently conducting Phase 3 trials of MDMA-assisted psychotherapy for PTSD—spanning eight research sites and hundreds of subjects.

Andrew Penn at the UCSF Medical School, has worn many hats in this work—as co-investigator, medical monitor, and study therapist. When I spoke with him in April 2023, the final participants in a MAPS study he was involved in had just completed their treatment (see the study under Mitchell et al. 2023). If results are favorable, MAPS will seek FDA approval for the prescription of MDMA, meaning patients with PTSD may have already been prescribed MDMA legally by the time you are reading this.

"It's been really interesting," Penn says, "to have a front-row seat at this ongoing research happening now all over the world."

Penn also described to me UCSF's role in Phase 2 trials of psilocybin-assisted psychotherapy for depression, sponsored by the Usona Institute, a nonprofit research institute exploring consciousness-expanding medicines. Such rigor is essential: only after safety and efficacy are conclusively established can we explore the creative and spiritual potential of these medicines.

THE GLARING GAP IN
END-OF-LIFE CARE

In initiating the first stage of the psychedelic renaissance, scientific researchers had to find a way to make psychedelics acceptable again. This meant first and foremost diminishing the government-created misperception of psychedelics as mere recreational drugs of abuse.

As Dr. Ira Byock, a palliative care specialist and author of *The Best Care Possible: A Physician's Quest to Transform Care Through the End of Life* (2012), warns, "These are not party drugs, damn it, and they're not rave drugs. . . . I'm afraid that in unsupervised hands, people who are using them for [the] wrong purpose can experience some very serious consequences."

Used appropriately in controlled settings, psychedelics show promise as revolutionary treatments. Byock is concerned that misused as recreational drugs, they remain potentially dangerous and perpetuate their taboo status. However, given the many millions of people who have used MDMA at raves, one might question Byock's worry.

In seeking to establish mainstream credibility, researchers took the same approach that worked with medical marijuana: focus first on the medicinal use, establish the safety and benefits, and broader acceptance will follow.

The same rationale likewise guided the decision to study MDMA for PTSD in veterans and first responders. If these treatments work for our heroes in uniform, how could we deny them to others?

Once people see the concrete alleviation of human suffering these treatments can bring about, public perception will begin to shift.

With psychedelic medicines, we start by pointing out how many people are suffering, and then ask, "Are we really going to deny an effective medicine to those in need?"

Modern medicine has made progress in managing physical suffering at the end of life, thanks to advancements in pain medications, palliative care, and hospice services. However, while we have learned to dull the body's agony, we still have few tools to soothe the anguish of the mind. Filling this hole was a strategic decision. If we wanted to change long-held misperceptions about psychedelics, we had to begin where the need was greatest.

As Anthony Bossis put it to me, "We really have a paucity of tools to help people with this existential, emotional, psychological angst, distress, and terror at the idea of this body and life ending."

This psychological and spiritual suffering represents one of the gaping holes in end-of-life care.

Those suffering from terminal illnesses represent a uniquely empathetic group, and their deep distress calls for deep interventions. By demonstrating the power of psychedelics to ease existential angst at life's end, we open the door for these substances to treat other forms of psychological suffering.

The story of Ernst Hilgard shows how taboo topics can derail careers. Like hypnosis for Hilgard, psychedelics were my forbidden fascination—their insights too radical for their times. However, after more than half a century of suppression by the U.S. government, the tide is finally beginning to turn.

Visionary scientists like Griffiths and Grob established solid reputations before wading into treacherous waters. Their trailblazing efforts reopened the portal to psychedelic research closed since the 1960s. Today, psychedelic studies are accelerating through FDA phases that assess safety, dosages, and benefits for conditions like PTSD, depression, and addiction. MDMA may get FDA approval soon for PTSD. Psilocybin looks promising for many uses. But this renaissance is still just beginning.

The old thinking is fading, but our work has just begun.

CHAPTER 3

Studies of Psychedelics for End-of-Life Distress

Proof of Safety and Efficacy

When I interviewed Lieutenant Sarko Gergerian, a Boston police officer and psychotherapist, on *Mind Body Health & Politics*, I found a kindred spirit. Like me, Gergerian's life was transformed by psychedelic experiences that forever changed the way he saw the world. In the 1960s, my eye-opening experiences with morning glory seeds and later LSD led me to take leave of my faculty position at the University of Michigan. I had the good fortune to live at the Esalen Institute in California during the 1967 "Summer of Love" in Northern California.

Gergerian had begun his career in the 1990s as a security guard for nightclubs and bars in Boston. He witnessed a significant change in the Boston nightclub scene when patrons switched from cocaine and alcohol to MDMA.

"The entire scene went from highly charged and dangerous people looking at each other like they were enemies to smiling faces in circles," he recounts during the interview. "People were welcoming and high-fiving and hugging each other."

I also know from experience how markedly different the effects of psychedelics are as compared to traditional party drugs like alcohol and cocaine, with the former tending to make people more cooperative and prosocial.

After twenty years as a security guard—Gergerian became a patrol officer with the police department in Winthrop, Massachusetts. In the meantime, he had also received a master's degree in psychology. The police chief started taking him to the International Association of Chiefs of Police (IACP) conference every year. This allowed Gergerian to attend supplementary classes, resiliency classes, and wellness classes. He then integrated the knowledge gained from these classes to improve the programs they had initiated in Winthrop, aiming to better serve the community and bridge the gap between law enforcement and the local residents.

"One year, the IACP was in Florida, and guess who was presenting at that conference?" Gergerian asks me.

It was my old friend Rick Doblin, founder of the Multidisciplinary Association for Psychedelic Studies.

In the conference flyer, it said "MDMA-Assisted Psychotherapy for Treatment-Resistant Severe PTSD." The word MDMA caught his eye.

"I had this lived experience from my work as a security guard—a front-row seat to the impact that this molecule has on people, on a scene, on culture," Gergerian explains.

"Now, here was this gentleman—Rick Doblin—presenting clinical trials about the efficacy of MDMA to help with treatment-resistant severe PTSD. I couldn't believe that this was happening at a chiefs of police conference."

That same day, Donald Trump was scheduled to speak at the conference during the same time slot as Rick, on the same floor of the convention hall.

"To the right is Donald Trump, and to the left is Rick Doblin," Gergerian recalls. "Thank goodness I went left, because they had given him and his crew a wonderful big room. They were probably expecting a lot of people to be interested in the topic, but there were only about fifteen of us in that room."

He sat down in the front row and listened to Rick explain the progress MAPS was making toward turning a Schedule I substance into a prescription medicine.

The results of MAPS' early studies blew him away.

"I couldn't believe it," he says.

"On that day, I learned that 67 percent of participants in the trial's phase no longer qualified for the PTSD diagnosis after undergoing MDMA-assisted psychotherapy using the MAPS protocol."

He repeats, "I couldn't believe it."

Lieutenant Gergerian was discovering what I had learned in the 1980s during my psychotherapy treatment with Dr. Robert Kantor in Atherton, California. Kantor administered MDMA to me during our sessions, which sparked my interest in researching its potential healing benefits. I met Rick in 1985, and we discussed the profound effects of MDMA on healing trauma. At that time, we were already aware of the molecule's efficacy in treating people with PTSD and other conditions. In 1985 MDMA was made illegal by the US government.

After Rick's talk ended, Gergerian was shaking with excitement. He jumped up on stage, and introduced himself.

"Rick asked me a few questions and found out that I was a working police officer and a psychotherapist. I said, 'How can I help you with this?' And he said, 'Become an MDMA-assisted psychotherapist,' and he gave me his card. When I reached out to him, I got into one of the first cohorts to be trained and then I was afforded access to a research protocol for 'healthy normals.'"

This Phase 2 MDMA trial for frontline responders, highlighted in the 2022 Netflix documentary *How to Change Your Mind*, played a pivotal role in altering Gergerian's outlook and life trajectory. His participation in the study, under a federally sanctioned research protocol, elicited profound emotional responses of love and gratitude, offering him a transformative perspective on the potential of MDMA-assisted therapy to address the challenges of severe, treatment-resistant PTSD. This trial, part of a series of studies conducted by the MAPS, aimed at exploring the therapeutic benefits of MDMA for individuals with PTSD, and underscored the significant promise of psychedelic-assisted therapy. The Phase 2 trials, which have been foundational in demonstrating the safety and efficacy of MDMA-assisted therapy, have paved the way for further research, including Phase 3 trials. These subsequent studies seek to consolidate MDMA-assisted therapy's standing as a potential treatment for PTSD, offering hope for frontline responders and others facing similar psychological burdens.

"My MDMA experience was federally sanctioned as part of a research protocol," Gergerian notes. "When the medicine took effect, I felt this deep overwhelming sense of love come across me. But what happened right after that sense of love was a sense of gratitude. It gave me the needed perspective as to how MDMA was going to help somebody that's struggling with treatment-resistant severe PTSD."

In addition to being one of the first police officers to legally undergo psychedelic-assisted psychotherapy, Gergerian earned certifications in addiction counseling, meditation instruction, and psychedelic-assisted psychotherapy. Gergerian has founded a "Guardian" policing model that uses peer support to help officers avoid job-related trauma. His story offers a glimpse into the promise of psychedelics to transform not only individuals but the systems in which they operate.

In law enforcement police officers tend to have a strong bias against "drug users." However perceptions are gradually changing regarding substances like psilocybin and MDMA with many former stereotypes starting to dissipate.

There is a great deal of second-hand anecdotal evidence now trickling into the popular perception, as more people become aware of the experiences of those who have experimented with psychedelic medicines, as opposed to other kinds of recreational drugs—and even pharmaceuticals.

In June of 2023 I presented at the MAPS-sponsored Psychedelic Science conference in Denver, Colorado. While there, I interviewed a group of police officers who were standing outside the Colorado Convention Center.

When asked about their sentiments regarding the psychedelic conference they said: "Every one of us has had a family member fucked up by Big Pharma medicines. If these people have something better to offer, we sure as hell are going to listen."

Anecdotal stories about the benefits of psychedelics are especially powerful coming from unexpected sources like a police lieutenant. But to break through the decades of misinformation and iron curtain

prohibition, hard data is needed to show the tangible medicinal benefits of psychedelics for specific conditions, such as end-of-life-distress.

ANECDOTAL DATA VS. DOUBLE-BLIND STUDIES

Like Gergerian, researchers at the forefront of psychedelic science are
building bridges between realms long divided. Stringent scientific meth-
odologies are being brought to bear on substances long considered taboo.
Double-blind, placebo-controlled trials represent the gold standard for
determining efficacy in medical research. These rigorous studies are the
only way to establish whether observed effects of any treatment are due
to the intervention itself, rather than to external factors like control
group dynamics or expectations of participants and researchers.

Double-blind studies require a significant amount of time, resources,
and oversight to execute properly. "Double-blind" means that neither
administrators nor subjects know who receives the active drug and who
receives the placebo until the trial is complete. This method controls for
the impact of experimenter biases on outcomes.

Of course, double-blind trials are not the only way to demonstrate
safety and efficacy. Anecdotal evidence, accumulated over time, also
deserves a great deal of credibility. To give an example from my own life,
hundreds of thousands of people have bathed in the medicinal waters
at the health sanctuary I created in 1972 at Wilbur Hot Springs. In
these past fifty years there have been no health department complaints.
Though not scientifically verified through double-blind experiments, it
is scientifically sound to consider the waters safe based on the hundreds
of thousands of 100 percent safe participants over the fifty-year period.

The same rationale applies to psychedelics. Millions have used
these substances in underground settings, yet emergency rooms report
a very small percentage of adverse events. However, as my British colleague Robin Carhart-Harris points out, it is essential to remember
that even a small percentage is a significant number of people when
applied to a large population. Thus as the number of psychedelic users
increases so will the number of people experiencing adverse effects. In
addition, any substance in the wrong hands or settings can be danger-

ous. We take important note that unlike heroin, cocaine, alcohol, or fentanyl, there have been no documented fatal overdoses from psilocybin or LSD.

While anecdotal evidence and personal experience have great meaning, robust data from clinical trials matter even more. We must not conflate the two or draw conclusions beyond what rigorous science can support. Long-term experience with psilocybin fosters confidence in its safety, but only gold-standard trials can demonstrate efficacy for medical use. We need evidence across populations to determine appropriate dosing, understand psychological effects, identify possible risks, and verify the benefits attributed to these substances.

Double-blind trials are not intended to replace wisdom accumulated through human experience over time. However, in an era when anything can be marketed with an anecdote, science serves as a bulwark against forces that would take advantage of public trust. Psychedelic medicines are too promising and too easily misused for us to lower our standards.

Some argue that the term "double-blind" is a misnomer when it comes to mind-altering substances like psychedelics, as the effects are typically conspicuous not only to participants who receive the actual psychedelic or the placebo but also to the researchers involved in the study, making it challenging to maintain the intended blindness.

As Don Lattin, the author of several books on psychedelics, including *The Harvard Psychedelic Club* (2010) and *God on Psychedelics* (2023), comments, "In a way, it's a joke because everybody knows who gets the placebo and who gets the real thing."

A New Yorker cartoon humorously touched on this conundrum by depicting a clinical trial with one group sitting placidly while the other dances deliriously, as in Henri Matisse's famous painting *The Dance*. The caption reads: "I guess we're the control group."

While blinding the experimental group may be challenging—their experience is unmistakable—the placebo group can be "naive," meaning they have never taken psychedelics before, thus allowing for the possibility of placebo effects. This is where double-blind placebo controls come in. The placebo effect is strong, and in therapy-based trials, the medication may only be secondary to the effects of the therapy.

Therefore, control groups are necessary to determine if perceived benefits are the result of the substance or therapy alone. For instance, three therapy sessions with a placebo may trigger positive changes, but are they equivalent to therapy plus psilocybin? Without control groups, we cannot know if the experimental group's response significantly differs from that of the control group.

In addition to using the gold standard, double-blind methodology, the studies on psychedelics for end-of-life distress to date have been carefully designed; from the substance dosage to patient screening, preparation, therapy sessions, and subsequent integration care.

SELECTING AND PREPARING PARTICIPANTS

In recent studies on psychedelic-assisted psychotherapy for end-of-life transitions, participants were required to have a diagnosis of anxiety, depression, or existential distress related to a terminal illness, most commonly cancer.

For example, Grob et al. (2011) screened patients with advanced-stage cancer who exhibited reactive anxiety, while Bossis selected patients with cancer-related anxiety and depression (Ross et al. 2016).

At NYU and Johns Hopkins, the focus has been on recruiting patients with life-threatening cancer who have a limited prognosis for survival. Exclusion criteria have typically been unstable medical conditions such as uncontrolled hypertension, as well as a history of or current psychotic spectrum illness (Ross et al. 2016; Griffiths et al. 2016).

As Bossis explains, "We look for people over twenty-one, English-speaking, with no history of psychosis or bipolar disorder—medically stable in terms of the cancer and its treatment—and presenting with anxiety, depression, hopelessness, or demoralization related to their diagnosis."

Before dosing, participants undergo preparatory sessions with their therapists. Grob conducted preparatory meetings to establish rapport and set the stage for the psilocybin experience. Bossis engaged in similar psychotherapy sessions to educate participants on what to expect and to discuss their intentions. Some patients had prior experience with psychedelics, others had never tried them before. Regardless of prior experience, preparation sessions aimed to provide a safe and supportive setting for all participants.

The preparation phase also allows therapists to screen for any psychological issues that may be exacerbated by psychedelics. As Grob explains, "We have seen a lot of psychopathology, and if we're paying attention, we get good at identifying it when we see it."

Proper screening and preparation minimizes adverse psychological reactions.

Gisele Fernandes-Osterhold, a psychotherapist at the California Institute for Integral Studies (CIIS), has been at the forefront of psychedelic research at the University of California San Francisco. She serves as the director of facilitation for several clinical trials on psilocybin at UCSF, including one on depression and anxiety in Parkinson's Disease (see Woolley 2021). Given these roles she has extensive experience preparing participants and guiding psychedelic sessions. Fernandes-Osterhold collaborates with UCSF's cutting-edge Translational Psychedelic Research (TrPR) Program, which studies how psychedelics impact the brain and mental health (Raison et al. 2023).

Reflecting on her experience preparing participants for psychedelic sessions, Fernandes-Osterhold explains:

> When a participant comes in, I prepare them for the journey. We have three preparatory sessions, each two hours long, where we look at their lives, who they are, how Parkinson's impacts their relationships, emotions, bodies, surroundings, and outlook—that's the qualitative aspect. And we prepare them in relationship to what a psychedelic experience can be. Some people who came through the studies were hippies in the sixties and seventies and had previous psychedelic experiences back in the day or in college. Others had no prior experience with psychedelics before the study. For everybody, we do the same preparation to discuss psilocybin—what it does in the body, psyche, thought processes, and the kinds of experiences one may encounter.

Fernandes-Osterhold tailors the preparation sessions to each participant, catering to those who are psychedelically naive as well as those who are experienced with psychedelics. She aims to provide a safe container and educate participants about the medicine's effects. This careful screening and rapport-building establishes trust prior to the psilocybin session.

In the studies on anxiety and depression, one or two therapists stay with the patient for safety and support during dosing sessions, which last four to six hours. Participants remain at the facility for some time after the effects have subsided to ensure safe reentry to daily life.

Well-trained guides are essential to the success and safety of psychedelic treatment. Their role is to help participants feel safe during the psilocybin experience without directing the participant's inner journey. Guides provide guidance if, and when, needed, while also allowing the medicine to work. Follow-up integration sessions help participants process their experiences and apply insights into daily living.

This careful screening, preparation, and therapeutic support provides the safety net for participants to navigate their psychedelic experience.

While a single dose of psilocybin can have a lasting impact, integration work consolidates these enduring changes.

The actual psychedelic experience is like entering one's personal gold mine. The follow-up integration sessions provide the opportunity to examine and polish the nuggets of gold taken from the mine.

CHOOSING PSILOCYBIN: SUBSTANCE AND DOSE

In all of these studies on end-of-life-distress, psilocybin was selected over other psychedelics like LSD or MDMA for several key reasons.

Duration of Action

The primary reason is psilocybin's shorter duration compared to LSD and some other psychedelic substances. As researcher Dr. Brian

Anderson explains, "Psilocybin's effects are shorter-acting than LSD, so a four- to six- hour experience is less taxing than eight to ten hours or longer."

This comment was echoed by Katherine MacLean, a writer and research scientist who did her postdoctoral research fellowship in psychopharmacology with Roland Griffiths at the Johns Hopkins University School of Medicine from 2009 to 2012.

"If you're showing up at eight o' clock in the morning at Hopkins for your psilocybin session, you can go home for dinner with your family," she notes.

Following her psilocybin study with Griffiths (MacLean, Johnson, and Griffiths 2011), MacLean was hired as a tenure-track faculty member in the Department of Psychiatry at Johns Hopkins. However, she left that position in 2013 after her younger sister's untimely death from cancer and traveled the world before settling on an organic farm with her husband.

In 2015, MacLean co-founded the Psychedelic Education and Continuing Care Program in New York and served as its inaugural director. There, she led training workshops and monthly integration groups focused on enhancing understanding and reducing the risks associated with psychedelic use.

When taking psychedelics which have a longer duration, the risks of an adverse effect can increase.

"If you're talking about LSD, it could last twelve hours for some people," she tells me in our first interview. "It's a very long journey. And if you're halfway through an LSD journey and you decide you don't like it, you've got a lot of territory to cover before you're back home."

Fewer Adverse Effects

Besides the duration, LSD also carries a higher risk of adverse psychological effects compared to psilocybin. According to Charles Grob, LSD is "more difficult to control and may be more likely than psilocybin to induce anxiety or paranoia."

Grob had also considered MDMA for end-of-life care but ultimately found psilocybin to be a more suitable medicine to work with in a clinical setting, as well as easier to get approval for.

"I had submitted a couple of protocols using MDMA that were not accepted," he tells me.

"In the late 90s, when we were submitting these protocols, there was a huge controversy over MDMA neurotoxicity. It was even suggested that young people who were taking MDMA were at risk of not only having serotonergic-related disorders, but also dopaminergic pathology such as Parkinson's disease."

Since the 90s, many of the concerns about MDMA's alleged neurotoxicity have been resolved. It turns out that the primary study, by Dr. George Ricaurte, on which these allegations of neurotoxicity were based, was later found to be seriously if not egregiously flawed. Despite the major inaccuracy of Ricaurte's results, they were presented to national politicians as factual. Consequently, the stigma attached to MDMA remains much stronger than the stigma surrounding psilocybin. Old prohibitions, even false ones, die hard.

Public Perception

LSD, like MDMA, carries a lingering and lasting stigma and controversy from the 1960s.

As Thomas Roberts, the academic and author of *Mindapps*, notes, "Imagine proposing LSD research to an Institutional Review Board whose knowledge comes only from politicians and media—it would severely damage the university's reputation." Therefore, the public stigma around LSD made psilocybin a more pragmatic choice.

Roberts further notes that psilocybin functions on the psyche in very similar ways as LSD, "You just need to take a larger dose to get the same effects."

"Psilocybin is harder to pronounce and spell than LSD," he adds. "I think that's part of the funny little difference."

Standardized Production

One downside of using psilocybin over pharmaceutical compounds like MDMA and LSD in clinical settings is that it's harder to standardize a dose, a requirement by the FDA, due to its natural occurrence in mushrooms.

This challenge was effectively addressed with the invention of synthetic psilocybin, enabling accurate, standardized dosing for research, unlike organic mushrooms with variable psilocybin concentrations. Nicholas Cozzi of the University of Wisconsin's Medical Center, and cofounder, along with Paul Daley, of the Alexander Shulgin Research Institute (where I serve as senior advisor), was authorized by the government to produce synthetic psilocybin.

Andrew Penn, a board-certified psychiatric nurse practitioner who helped oversee the psilocybin study out of UCSF, explains, "The FDA would not allow ground-up mushrooms due to their variance in psilocybin content. Much like different strains of cannabis have varying degrees of THC, CBD, and the other cannabinoids, there is considerable variance in how much psilocybin is in an actual fungal fruiting body of the mushroom" (Daws et al. 2022). For pragmatic and scientific reasons, synthetic psilocybin emerged as the optimal psychedelic to rigorously study the context of end-of-life distress.

DOSING

Over the years, studies involving cancer patients have compared a range of psilocybin doses to balance between safety and efficacy. Grob and colleagues used a cautious moderate dose of 0.2 milligrams per kilogram of body weight in their pioneering 2011 study (Grob et al. 2011). For a 150-pound person, this equates to around 13.6 milligrams of psilocybin.

Bossis and his team administered a slightly higher dose of 0.3 milligrams per kilogram body weight (Ross et al. 2016). So for a 150-pound person, this would be 20.5 milligrams of psilocybin.

Griffiths and colleagues (2016) compared low doses of 1–3 milligrams per 70 kilograms of body weight to high doses of 22–30 milligrams per 70 kilograms. The high dose of 22–30 milligrams equals approximately 3–4 grams of dried mushrooms for an average adult.

For context, according to the famed psychedelic explorer Terence

McKenna, 5 grams of dried mushrooms was considered a "heroic dose." With average psilocybin levels of around 1 percent in dried mushrooms, this equals about 50 milligrams of psilocybin. McKenna believed that a heroic dose of mushrooms could reliably bring about the experience known as ego death or ego dissolution, in which a person's sense of identity with their physical body and other identity markers fades into a kind of cosmic consciousness or unity with the universe.

The studies here referenced aimed to use doses high enough to elicit clinically meaningful effects while minimizing the risk of severely challenging psychological experiences.

Starting with lower doses helped establish safety before gradually increasing the dose to identify the ideal therapeutic range.

While the milligram amounts appear small, psilocybin is highly potent even at levels below a "heroic dose." As MacLean notes, with psilocybin, "It's not a chemical effect alone, it's the context plus the chemistry" that determines the experience.

The environment and mindset, or "set and setting" are critical variables along with the substance and dosage. Preparation sessions help patients feel safe, guided, and ready to surrender to the experience. The therapists' compassionate presence and subsequent follow-up are vital for helping patients actualize insights.

The rigorous dose-response analysis has enabled researchers to determine dosage guidelines specifically for clinically supervised settings. Weight-correlated lower doses of 10–15 milligrams may provide a gentler introduction to psilocybin, moderate doses around 20 milligrams balance safety and efficacy for many, and doses up to 30 milligrams appear to enhance mystical-type experiences that may help patients find new meaning and confront their anxiety related to death.

While challenging to define scientifically, the qualitative shifts in consciousness may be key to psilocybin's therapeutic potential. This raises the question of how subjective mystical experiences can be quantified and recognized as "tangible medical benefits" to warrant legal medical use.

MEASURING OUTCOMES

The studies use various psychometric scales to assess the psychological effects of psilocybin treatment both during sessions and throughout the follow-up period.

The most well-known tools is the Mystical Experience Questionnaire (MEQ), created in 1962 by Dr. Walter Pahnke, the physician and minister at Harvard's Divinity School who was responsible for the now famous "Good Friday Experiment." The original 39-item MEQ aimed to quantify the mystical-type experiences that researchers hypothesized were linked to significant psychological transformations.

Bossis explains, the MEQ measures key aspects of mystical experience including "a sense of unity with all things, a sense of sacredness or humility, encountering ultimate reality that speaks with profound authority, and the ineffability of transcending normal time and space."

In the 1970s, psychedelic science pioneer Bill Richards reduced the MEQ to thirty statements that participants rate on a scale from "not at all" to "extreme." This simplified version provides numerical scores for each dimension of the mystical experience.

> Instructions: Looking back on the entirety of your psilocybin session, please rate the degree to which at any time during that session you experienced the following phenomena. Answer each question according to your feelings, thoughts, and experiences at the time of the psilocybin session. In making each of your ratings, use the following scale (MacLean 2012):

- 0 — none (not at all)
- 1 — so slight cannot decide
- 2 — slight
- 3 — moderate
- 4 — strong (equivalent in degree to any other strong experience)
- 5 — extreme (more than any other time in my life and stronger than 4)

1. Freedom from the limitations of your personal self and feeling a unity or bond with what was felt to be greater than your personal self.
2. Experience of pure being and pure awareness (beyond the world of sense impressions).
3. Experience of oneness in relation to an "inner world" within.
4. Experience of the fusion of your personal self into a larger whole.
5. Experience of unity with ultimate reality.
6. Feeling that you experienced eternity or infinity.
7. Experience of oneness or unity with objects and/or persons perceived in your surroundings.
8. Experience of the insight that "all is One."
9. Awareness of the life or living presence in all things.
10. Gain of insightful knowledge experienced at an intuitive level.
11. Certainty of encounter with ultimate reality (in the sense of being able to "know" and "see" what is really real at some point during your experience.
12. You are convinced now, as you look back on your experience, that in it you encountered ultimate reality (i.e., that you "knew" and "saw" what was really real).
13. Sense of being at a spiritual height.
14. Sense of reverence.
15. Feeling that you experienced something profoundly sacred and holy.
16. Experience of amazement.
17. Feelings of tenderness and gentleness.
18. Feelings of peace and tranquility.
19. Experience of ecstasy.
20. Sense of awe or awesomeness.
21. Feelings of joy.
22. Loss of your usual sense of time.
23. Loss of your usual sense of space.
24. Loss of usual awareness of where you were.

25. Sense of being "outside of" time, beyond past and future.
26. Being in a realm with no space boundaries.
27. Experience of timelessness.
28. Sense that the experience cannot be described adequately in words.
29. Feeling that you could not do justice to your experience by describing it in words.
30. Feeling that it would be difficult to communicate your own experience to others who have not had similar experiences.

As Bossis notes, "The MEQ has held up remarkably well for sixty years now in capturing the qualitative nature of these experiences."

His team used a version of the MEQ revised by Griffiths at Johns Hopkins.

Griffiths's early studies found a clear link between higher MEQ scores and greater reductions in cancer-related distress.

As Bossis sums up, "Those who had the mystical experience, as measured by the MEQ, had a higher degree of reduction in depression, anxiety, hopelessness, and demoralization."

This aligns with my own experience. While transcendent states can arise through activities like love or nature, nothing compares to the unity, sacredness, and ineffability occasioned by high-dose psychedelics.

Bossis also notes that an experience can still be therapeutic without classical mysticism: "People can revisit their lives, resolve conflicts, feel forgiveness and love. Those outcomes don't need to be only in this mystical dimension."

Yet, MEQ data suggests that the mystical dimension is key to psilocybin's efficacy. Griffiths's 2016 follow-up study found a lasting decrease in depression and anxiety, along with improvement in quality of life, meaning, and optimism fourteen months after a single psilocybin dose—primarily for those who had scored high on the MEQ. Beyond the MEQ, researchers have used other scales to assess different facets of the psychedelic experience. For example, the Death Transcendence Scale (Hood and Morris 1983) measures how individuals perceive death, while the Purpose in Life Scale (Robbins and Francis 2000) measures a person's sense of meaning in life. These measures aim to quantify complex subjective experiences in terms the FDA can recognize as "tangible medical benefits." Nonetheless, some nuance is undoubtedly lost in translation. We lack language for fully conveying the profound essence of these experiences.

The accumulated data has established clear correlations between psilocybin's effects on different psychometric scales and lasting relief from end-of-life distress. These pioneering studies make a compelling case for psilocybin's safety and efficacy when administered in controlled settings.

Group Therapy: The Future of Psychedelic Medicine?

In 1968, after leaving the University of Michigan to pursue a career outside academia, I established a clinic in San Francisco called the Gestalt Institute for Multiple Psychotherapy. The name was somewhat confusing, but its meaning was that two therapists were present in every therapy session, a technique I adopted from the pioneering Atlanta Psychiatric Clinic, led by Drs. Carl Whitaker and John Walkington. They were doing innovative work in psychotherapy and the multiple-therapist-tactic was shown to be profoundly effective—and far more so than what a single therapist could achieve.

Nowadays, institutions such as Johns Hopkins and NYU are using the same two-therapist protocol in their psychedelic research. This extra precaution is perceived as a particularly safe approach by the government and Institutional Review Boards (IRBs). However, in my opinion, this model will prove impractical and too expensive in the long-term, as it did at my clinic. It was too costly to have two doctors present in the same room with one patient. This would have meant treating only the super-wealthy, which did not align with my political beliefs.

A clinical trial by Dr. Manish Agrawal at the Aquilino Cancer Center in Maryland investigated the feasibility of using a group therapy model to reduce the costs associated with multiple therapists in each session. The study was conducted in partnership with mental health company 'Compass Pathways'—which, in 2018, received

FDA breakthrough therapy designation for psilocybin therapy for treatment-resistant depression. (This study is the one mentioned in the Compass Pathways 2021 citation in the reference list.)

The Healing Center at the Aquilino Cancer Center was specifically designed with four rooms for psilocybin therapy and an observation area for the lead therapist to facilitate the group therapy model. This allows four patients to be treated by five therapists instead of requiring eight therapists for four subjects, as in traditional protocols. According to Dr. Agrawal, this approach provides not only savings in terms of therapist hours but also therapeutic benefits as patients going through cancer treatment in groups often develop a sense of community and support each other's recovery journey.

The study at Aquilino aims to rigorously evaluate the group therapy model both clinically and economically. If the protocol is approved by regulators, it could significantly expand access to psychedelic therapy by reducing the costs of multiple individual therapists required for each session.

INITIAL RESULTS: A FEASIBLE AND MEANINGFUL APPROACH

To date, cancer studies have demonstrated that psilocybin combined with psychotherapy can significantly—and durably—reduce end-of-life distress.

For example, Grob's 2011 pilot study involving twelve patients with advanced cancer represents an early effort to reestablish psilocybin's safety. With a moderate dose of 0.2 milligrams of psilocybin per kilogram of body weight, Grob found no serious adverse events linked to psilocybin.

On self-reported psychological measures, Grob found trends toward diminished anxiety and depressive symptoms persisting weeks to months after treatment in the psilocybin group compared to the placebo group. For instance, on the Beck Depression Inventory, psilocybin patients' scores decreased by almost 30 percent from the first session to one month after the second session. These effects did not reach statistical significance due to the study's small sample size but hinted at therapeutic potential.

On the State-Trait Anxiety Inventory, Grob found no significant changes in state anxiety, but a statistically significant decrease in longer-term trait anxiety following psilocybin treatment. This decrease in a more enduring anxiety measure suggests reduction in stress levels over time.

Eleven of the twelve subjects reported mood boosts following their psilocybin session. Though not statistically significant, participants also showed improved mood up to two weeks after psilocybin treatment on the Profile of Mood States assessment.

While most of these psychological effects were subtle and not statistically significant—potentially due to its modest dose—this pilot study succeeded as an initial proof of safety—the first step in revisiting psilocybin's clinical promise. Without demonstrated safety and acceptability for patients, interest in psychedelic therapy could have stalled. However, by providing a framework for safe administration, Grob helped pave the way for the more decisive trials that followed.

More robust evidence came from Griffiths's 2016 double-blind trial of fifty-one cancer patients. A single high dose of psilocybin, approximately 22 to 30 milligrams per 70 kilograms, produced large, significant decreases in measures of depression, anxiety, and existential distress related to the cancer diagnosis, with effects lasting over six months for most patients. For instance, five weeks after the psilocybin session, 92 percent of patients showed significant improvement in depression symptoms versus only 32 percent after the very low dose (which was 1 to 3 milligrams per 70 kilograms). These response rates stayed remarkably high at 79 percent after six months.

Similarly, six months later, 65 percent of the high-dose group achieved remission of depressed mood to normal levels. This is remarkable given that only around 35 percent of advanced cancer patients normally achieve remission of depression with standard antidepressants.

The high-dose group also reported reductions exceeding 50 percent in anxiety, demoralization, hopelessness, and fear of death.

Improvements in quality of life and optimism were similarly substantial and enduring.

Griffiths's study suggests that psilocybin's mystical qualities may play a crucial role in facilitating these benefits. Those rating their experience as "very mystical" showed the greatest improvements in attitudes, mood, and behavior. Staying blind to conditions, Griffiths obscured the dosage levels, suggesting his results were attributable to psilocybin's effects rather than mere expectations by either the researchers or the participants.

Likewise, in the 2016 double-blind trial by Bossis and Ross of twenty-nine cancer patients, a single moderate dose of psilocybin rapidly improved symptoms of anxiety and depression in most participants, with benefits lasting over six months. The dose was approximately 0.3 milligrams per kilogram of body weight—far less than the high doses used in Griffiths' study. Yet, this moderate dose still resulted in substantial reductions in anxiety, depression, and cancer-related existential distress. Eighty-three percent of the psilocybin group showed significant improvement in depression symptoms just seven weeks after treatment, compared to only 14 percent of the placebo group. These response rates remained at approximately 60–80 percent even six and a half months later. While limited by sample size, this study showed that even moderate doses of psilocybin in combination with psychotherapy can durably improve cancer-related distress.

Beyond quantifiable symptoms, Ross and his researchers (2016) found participants in the psilocybin group rated the experience as among the most meaningful and spiritually significant of their lives, with over half deeming it the single most meaningful experience. This further cements the proposition that the mystical phenomena described by participants may have played a key role in psilocybin's therapeutic benefits. Similar to the findings in Griffiths' study, the intensity of patients' mystical experience correlated with and predicted their reductions in anxiety and depression. The treatment was safe, rapidly effective, and provided profound personal meaning for participants.

In 2018, Anderson conducted an open-label pilot study exploring psilocybin-assisted group therapy for fifteen demoralized, gay-identified men with HIV (Human Immunodeficiency Virus), marking the first modern trial combining psilocybin with group therapy. By initiating rigorous research on psilocybin group therapy, Anderson broadened our understanding of safe administration protocols beyond individual settings. Participants received individual psilocybin sessions within an eleven-week span of group therapy. The psilocybin doses ranged from 22 to 32 mg, averaging 27 mg (Anderson et al. 2020).

Anderson found the intervention to be relatively safe, with no serious adverse reactions attributable to psilocybin. However, there was a high rate of expected, transient anxiety reactions, with eight participants experiencing moderate or severe anxiety during their sessions.

On the primary outcome of demoralization, Anderson observed significant improvements from baseline to the end of treatment at a three-month follow-up. For instance, approximately 50 percent of participants showed more than 50 percent reduction in demoralization at the end of treatment.

Furthermore, Anderson observed reductions in symptoms of depression, grief, and PTSD.

However, not all observed effects could be measured through the assessment tools used in the study. "There were things in some of their lives that changed in ways we didn't capture in our measures," Anderson says. "For instance, some overcame shame about their diagnosis, became more socially connected, or showed reduced anxiety."

Through careful screening and support, Anderson demonstrated the feasibility of combining psilocybin with group therapy for complex patient demographics. Limitations like small sample size notwithstanding, the results indicate psilocybin group therapy's potential as a more cost-effective model than individual psilocybin-assisted psychotherapy while providing meaningful experiences and benefits comparable to individual treatment.

With careful design and oversight, alternative models could help address access barriers while maintaining high safety standards. The progress made in psychedelic science thus far is historic. But has it reached a tipping point yet beyond reversal, or might the door slam shut again?

PAST THE TIPPING POINT?

Anderson hopes that conventional allopathic psychiatry will continue to learn from traditional settings where psychoactive plants and psychedelics have been used for hundreds of thousands of years to heal people.

"I'm optimistic we can find ways to incorporate this sometimes radical type of care into conventional settings," he says. "I'm certainly more hopeful about how we can find ways to make psychedelic healing fit into conventional settings and do that in respectful and safe ways."

The progress has been astonishing—and frankly, surprising. For those of us who have long fought for this research to become a reality, there is concern that the doors might slam shut again at any moment.

Bossis recalled that even after FDA and DEA approval, he and his team were still whispering among their colleagues. "You didn't talk about this for fear of how it would be perceived," he tells me.

Each study had to prove safety anew before proceeding to the next phase.

Yet, in recent years, regulatory bodies have generally shown their support.

"What they want to see is safety and efficacy—primarily safety," Bossis explains. "That was being shown in the Hopkins and UCLA trials, so there was a foundation to stand upon. Then, our trial showed safety as well. It was a new era that was beginning."

For those battle-scarred from past campaigns, each step forward still feels precarious—as if the rug might be pulled out from under us at any moment. But the younger generation of researchers, who did not live through the long suppression, sees more promise of permanent progress.

Anderson told me that the parts of the federal and state government entities he interacts with are "open and encouraging to those conducting scientific work that benefits public health." He pointed to the fact that UCSF even has an FDA contract to study underground psychedelic groups and share lessons on safety.

"I interpret that as evidence that much of the federal government, or at least the parts that I interact with, recognize the need to learn more about implementing this well and safely," Anderson elaborates. "They want to understand what's happening in these underground groups so we can figure out the best practices for incorporating psychedelics into regulated settings moving forward."

Anderson even sees the potential to initiate studies within state-regulated facilities in states such as Oregon, Colorado, and California, as they are currently in the process of legalizing and decriminalizing psychedelics.

Perhaps the optimism of the new generation is right. The scientific rigor of today's research is unparalleled; the therapeutic potential undeniable. If we follow the data where it leads, these treatments are likely to establish a place in mainstream healthcare. It seems the genie might indeed be out of the bottle for good.

CHAPTER 4

Mechanism of Action

How Psychedelics Help the Dying Overcome End-of-Life Distress

My first experience with psychedelics as a graduate student in Michigan changed my understanding of life and death forever. In the midst of my journey, after ingesting the four hundred heavenly blue morning glory seeds, which I mentioned earlier in this book, I saw what seemed like my own spirit leave my body and float out into space. There, in the inky blackness, was a strange shape that shouldn't have been strictly possible in three dimensions: a flat, pink strip, twisting and turning back in on itself. I recognized the configuration of my vision as a Möbius strip: a continuous shape with only one surface and one edge.

Floating along this never-ending ribbon were spheres of light—souls, I somehow understood—cycling through the universe. At times, droplets broke from this stream, falling to Earth where they took a new form as life. I watched, stunned, as the boundaries between mind and matter dissolved. It seemed in that moment all separateness converged in an eternal flow.

My vision of oneness with other souls in the universe took on new meaning and importance. I viewed this vision through the eyes of my training as a clinical psychologist, asking how insights gained outside the functioning of everyday consciousness might be applied to a world in need of healing. My task has been to follow this path.

In the years that followed my initial experience, I learned that many others encountered similar visions. Psychedelics seem to reliably provide experiences of unity, ego transcendence, and dissolved boundaries that are extremely difficult to capture in words. The world of art, such as the paintings of Alex Gray—showing humans as electrochemical magnetic beings—come closer to describing the psychedelic experience than word descriptions or scientific papers. Yet, from scientific research we learn that these mystical experiences translate into clinically significant benefits, as highlighted by the research trials discussed in the previous chapter.

In studies involving patients facing death, psychedelic-assisted psychotherapy led to marked decreases in anxiety, depression, and distress. For direct comparison, 83 percent of cancer patients showed clinically significant reductions in depression seven weeks after a single psilocybin dose at NYU (Ross et al. 2016), and an impressive 92 percent after an initial high dose in the study at Johns Hopkins (Griffiths 2016). Such outcomes are virtually unprecedented utilizing conventional pharmaceutical medications alone.

The mechanisms behind psychedelics' success where traditional treatments and medications have not provided relief are becoming clearer to me, thanks to my personal tutors—the distinguished guests I interviewed for my book *Psychedelic Wisdom: The Astonishing Rewards of Mind Altering Substances*. The individuals in *Psychedelic Wisdom* had the courage to speak publicly about their personal experiences with psychedelics as well as, in some cases, their groundbreaking research.

HOW DO PSYCHEDELICS ALLEVIATE END-OF-LIFE-DISTRESS?

Psychedelics differ from many traditional medications in a fundamental way: they act primarily upon the mind. The word *psychedelic* means "soul manifesting" or "mind manifesting." Psychedelic medications create experiences that transform one's sense of self, connection to others, and understanding of existence.

As Anthony Bossis explains:

> Psychedelics draw us into consciousness in a way that [introduces] existentially oriented landscapes. They surface themes around impermanence, death, rebirth, grief . . . [and] recalibrating with matters profoundly meaningful for the dying.

Bossis believes that these medicines have particular power of transformational healing in those near the end of life:

> For the person whose body is about to stop working . . . this transcendent experience pulls the lens back . . . and helps them see themselves in a . . . larger landscape. It has the capacity to recalibrate suffering.
>
> When a certain experience is achieved, we're seeing better outcome levels in . . . end-of-life distress. Why would that be? What is it about consciousness that has this . . . spiritual essence?

This connection between transcendent experiences and healing remains mysterious, yet undeniable.

Beyond subjective experiences, there is also a concrete neurobiological basis for the antidepressant and anxiolytic effects of psilocybin.

Animal studies show that serotonergic psychedelics like psilocybin reduce anxiety. Rodent trials have found decreased anxiety behaviors after administering psychedelics, and modifying serotonin receptors in rodent brains affected anxiety levels, suggesting psilocybin's anxiolytic benefits may relate to changes in serotonin signaling.

In humans, differences in serotonin receptor density in certain brain regions correlate with anxiety symptoms. Thus, psilocybin may rapidly and durably reduce anxiety by downregulating particular serotonin-receptor subtypes.

Several lines of evidence implicate serotonin receptors in depression: postmortem studies show elevated cortical serotonin receptor levels in depressed suicide victims. Receptor density decreases after sustained antidepressant treatment. Furthermore, psilocybin enhances glutamate transmission and increases activity of cortical α-amino-3-hydroxy-5-methyl-4-isoxazoleproprionic acid (AMPA) receptors, which stimulates production of Brain-Derived Neurotropic Factor (BDNF), a protein linked to nerve growth and plasticity. The upregulation of AMPA and BDNF, known for their roles in antidepressant responses, may underlie the therapeutic benefits of psilocybin.

Recent research also highlights alterations in the medial prefrontal cortex and connectivity in the "default mode network," areas linked to depression through their hyperactivity and connectivity. The so-called default mode network represents a neurological basis for ego and self-reflection, offering insights into psychedelics' mechanism of action. The default mode network (DMN) is a large-scale brain network that becomes active when a person is not focused on the outside world and the brain is at wakeful rest, such as during daydreaming and mind-wandering. It is also active when individuals are thinking about others, thinking about themselves, remembering the past, and planning for the future. The DMN includes the medial prefrontal cortex, posterior cingulate cortex, and angular gyrus. Research has shown that psychedelic substances can dramatically reduce the activity and connectivity of the DMN. This reduction is thought to underlie the profound alterations in sense of self, ego dissolution, and the experience of unity that often characterize the psychedelic state. The DMN's usual activity patterns are disrupted, allowing for a more unconstrained style of cognition. This temporary disruption of the DMN may allow individuals to break free from rigid, habitual patterns of thought and behavior, potentially facilitating perspective shifts and psychological insight.

Moreover, the long-term effects of psychedelics on the DMN are of great interest in the context of treating mental health conditions. Studies have shown that the DMN is hyperactive and hyperconnected in conditions like depression, leading to excessive rumination and self-focus. The ability of psychedelics to reset the activity patterns of the DMN may underlie their potential as rapid-acting antidepressants and anxiolytics. The so-called default mode network represents a neurological basis for ego and self-reflection, offering insights into psychedelics' mechanism of action. Thanks to new fMRI technology we can now see changes in the default mode network's activity.

Jahan Khamsehzadeh, author of *The Psilocybin Connection*, described studies to me showing that the DMN is overactive in anxiety and depression:

> In terms of neurology, what we see is what we call the default mode network in the brain that activates when we think of the ego self, the "I-I-I," "me-me-me." So, focus acts as a repressive function for the rest of our brain.
>
> The default mode network is overly dense in people with anxiety and depression. If you're constantly in pain and somebody's pinching you, you can't help but think of that pain and think of yourself. The whole brain begins to hyperconnect.
>
> The ego self is like a very loud voice that represses all the other voices inside. Once that quiets down and the person is relaxed, at peace, and feeling safe, all the subconscious and unconscious factors rise. So, what we tend to see is a unified experience within the brain that correlates with the unified experience people are having within themselves, with the environment, and with the cosmos.

My only problem with this explanation is that the term 'default mode network' applies computer lingo to human experiences. The term is too general to capture the depth of psychedelic insights, reflecting a comprehensive approach affecting the physical, neurophysiological, mental, energetic, and symbolic dimensions of a person's being.

Outcomes, as Khamsehzadeh notes, depend on "how [the patient] is making meaning . . . recreating narratives of self, life, and re-engagement."

Gisele Fernandes-Osterhold shares my skepticism about attempts to boil down the essence of the mystical experience to changes in the firing of different neurons or regions of the brain. She says:

[Some researchers] are mostly interested in decreased default mode network activity, decreased prefrontal cortex activity, or the serotonergic system of the brain. There are professionals from different medical fields investigating the psychopharmacological mechanisms through which psilocybin produces long-term alterations in cortical networks. But I want to believe it's a holistic treatment. While we investigate the physical and neurophysiological aspects, we ought to be very interested in the body, mind, energy, meaning, symbols, and all that encompasses a person in that moment in life and how they're making meaning of that experience and recreating their narratives about who they are, what life is, and how they want to re-engage in life. I don't believe it's purely biochemical.

Gisele believes that a fundamental shift in consciousness occurs when a patient has a profound experience with psychedelics:

The German philosopher Heidegger differentiated between our two modes of existence: the everyday mode and the ontological mode. We go about our lives living in an everyday mode with our ordinary consciousness, preoccupied about things, and going about choices and relationships in a certain way.

When something big happens to us—like a threatening disease, a breakup, loss of a loved one, or sometimes through a dream—there can be an opportunity to switch that everyday mode into an ontological mode. He [Heidegger] talked about the ontological mode as the miracle of being.

It's almost like reality shifts right in front of us in the face of an irreversible experience, and it awakens us out of this everyday mode. It's as though the curtain closes and then a new scene comes on.

I tend to think about those moments as a confrontation with death. When we get in touch with pain—when we face suffering and we go through it—there's a possibility of transformation.

The key, it seems, goes beyond biochemistry alone.

PROBING THE MYSTICAL EXPERIENCE

For researchers seeking publishable results, the Mystical Experience Questionnaire (MEQ) provides a quantitative assessment tool to correlate with improvement in symptoms based on the subjective strength of the psychedelic experience.

Psychedelics defy reductionist explanations; their effects ripple across dimensions—physiological, psychological, symbolic, and spiritual. They dissolve accustomed ways of understanding self and world, occasioning new ones of profound, yet elusive significance.

Psilocybin gives people a strong sense of connection with other human beings and the planet. With over two hundred species of psilocybin mushrooms sharing the same mind-altering active ingredient, I asked Khamsehzadeh why this particular mushroom has such positive effects and what the mechanisms are that foster such positivity and sense of connection. This is what he told me:

> In years of looking at it, I've found some very good answers, and yet some part remains a great mystery.
>
> If we look at psilocybin itself, it grows out of the fungi kingdom, which has been around for about 2.5 billion years. We're talking about the organisms that created the soil for all of the biosphere to evolve. Our entire evolutionary trajectory has been on top of this living network.
>
> In this intelligent, complex network that unites all the plants in the environment is the mushroom—the cap and stem formation. When ingested, psilocybin, the active ingredient in psychedelic mushrooms, docks onto the 5-HT_{2A} serotonin receptors in our brain, creating hyperconnected brain states and expanding our consciousness and creating a sense of ecological awakening and empathy with all of the environment.
>
> I believe these compounds grow in the ecosystem to regulate consciousness. Just as our body has hormones and compounds that create a state of homeostasis, the ecosystem tries to do the same. We are partly drawing from Gaia hypothesis—the idea that there are

chemicals in the environment that attempt to regulate all organisms. This helps us see how deeply intelligent and interconnected we are with all of life.

James Lovelock's Gaia hypothesis proposes that Earth operates as a self-regulating system, where living (biotic) and non-living (abiotic) factors interact to sustain environmental conditions conducive to life. The hypothesis suggests that Earth behaves as a single organism, with each component interacting and influencing one another to maintain an equilibrium. As the name implies, it is a speculative *hypothesis*—not a confirmed proposition. You will not see the term referenced in any of the scientific literature on the medicinal benefits of the psilocybe mushroom.

You also do not need to subscribe to any particular religious or mystical beliefs to have a profound experience of renewed meaning in your life.

"THE GRATEFUL DEAD," PSYCHEDELICS, AND SPIRITUALITY

The iconic psychedelic rock band Grateful Dead fostered an entire spiritual, almost religious, subculture around their music, which served as a soundtrack for psychedelic exploration. Their name itself hints at the transcendent states their concerts helped to induce.

I once discussed with religious scholar Christian Greer the meaning behind Grateful Dead's unusual moniker. As you may recall, during my first psychedelic experience, I experienced ego death, the dissolution of the ordinary sense of self. Fortunately, I recognized it as a passing state of consciousness rather than believing I was literally dying. Afterward, I felt immense gratitude for having glimpsed reality unencumbered by ego.

Greer notes that "surrendering the ego and becoming grateful to undergo ego death" represents a core teaching of psychedelic wisdom. The perfect psychedelic community, he proposed, would be a group happily freed from ego's constraints, living communally beyond conditioned worldviews. (From what I hear from Mariavittoria Mangini, the Hog Farm, in Laytonville, California, may be such a place.)

The Acid Tests conducted by novelist Ken Kesey in the 1960s introduced thousands to psychedelic culture through the music of the Grateful Dead. Their cryptic lyrics became guideposts for navigating these altered states of consciousness. Even an institutional support system emerged, with medical tents at concerts to assist people during difficult trips. "Deadhead" communities cultivated and passed down techniques for safe psychedelic exploration.

Though the original members have aged, the Grateful Dead's legacy persists through new generations of fans and cover bands. As Greer noted, the internet itself emerged from early networks sharing recordings of Grateful Dead shows. The name and music of the Grateful Dead seeded teachings on ego transcendence that have taken root through decades of spiritual seekers. Even now, the Grateful Dead's ethos continues redefining religion for the psychedelic age, building communities around surrendering the ego's grip.

EGO DISSOLUTION

Ego dissolution refers to the loss of one self identity and a sense of merging with everything on the planet, or perhaps in the universe. It is a realization of the smallness of each of us and at the same time of the connectedness with everything. Ego dissolution is often experienced as a peak experience. Ego death, on the other hand, is experienced as though it is a real death, for one goes through a subjective feeling of dying, and then, of course, one comes to realize it was simply a major impactful experience with coming to grips with the fear of death.

Peter Sjöstedt-Hughes, a philosopher at the University of Exeter and author of the book *Noumenautics: Metaphysics–Meta-Ethics–Psychedelics*, emphasizes the importance of precision when discussing alleged mystical experiences. He believes in drilling down into definitions and historical understandings of the term *mystical experience* to gain a deeper understanding of it.

His belief is that not all psychedelic experiences are mystical. "One of the four criteria the English philosopher Bertrand Russell used to define mysticism was to go beyond good and evil, by which he meant to go beyond one's ideology and see it from above," he says.

Sjöstedt-Hughes's groundbreaking 2021 book, *Modes of Sentience: Psychedelics, Metaphysics, Panpsychism*, includes a quote from the social critic and philosopher Herbert Marcuse about the psychedelic experience. In his 1969 *Essay on Liberation*, Marcuse observes, "The 'trip' involves the dissolution of the ego shaped by the established society—an artificial and short-lived dissolution. But the artificial and 'private' liberation anticipates, in a distorted manner, an exigency of the social liberation: the revolution must be at the same time a revolution in perception which will accompany the material and intellectual reconstruction of society, creating the new aesthetic environment. Awareness of the need for such a revolution in perception, for a new sensorium, is perhaps the kernel of truth in the psychedelic search."

Sjöstedt-Hughes interprets Marcuse to be saying that the psychedelic experience gives a person a completely new perspective—not only on themselves, but on society at large. "You see yourself and society or politics in a new light, one that you perhaps never imagined before, because of course, psychedelics can push you far beyond imagination," Sjöstedt-Hughes says.

I relate to this, based on my own first psychedelic experience, which set me on a mission to make these medicines and this experience available for all—so that we might recognize our interconnectedness and no longer live as if competition and winning were the end goal.

My sense of fearlessness in the face of both death and social pressure to avoid taboo topics arose out of my numerous 'close encounters' with the other side—both psychedelic experiences of metaphysical "ego death" and actual near-death experiences in which I actually came close to dying.

A near-death experience (NDE) is a profound psychological event that occurs to a person close to death or in situations of intense physical or emotional danger, such as my motorcycle accidents. My experience of floating outside my body in darkness is a common attribute in near-death experiences, along with the stereotypical "bright light at the end of a tunnel."

Some people who come back from near-death experiences report having communicated with deceased loved ones. I did not experience either the bright light or communicate with the departed, but I did hear a voice telling me that I could still make a difference, which in turn ended up making a critical difference in my own decision to strive for my life.

Once again, science to this date has no way to confirm the validity of these supernatural-sounding accounts in material terms, but we can discuss the tangible effects they have on the person when they return to "this world."

Bossis told me that around 10–20 percent of people who undergo near-death experiences have mystical experiences similar to those who participate in his studies on the effects of psychedelics on end-of-life distress.

"They're dissimilar in some ways, but the values are the same in the sense of love, connection, and no fear when they come back to consciousness," Bossis says.

"That effect is sustained. People with NDEs, for the rest of their life, seem to be less afraid. I think if these experiences are had earlier in life, that ideally would help someone recalibrate with a greater sense of equanimity walking through this incredible life, where people are often crippled with fear of the end."

There would seem to be some commonalities between near-death experiences, "ego death," and actual death. Witnessing the inevitability of death, directly experiencing it, dramatically reduces culture-induced anxiety and fear.

Sjöstedt-Hughes speculates that this new outlook on society's hypocrisy might be why psychedelics have been perceived as such a threat. "I do think that is a power of psychedelics and perhaps one of many reasons why they are prohibited," he says.

If people stop fearing death, they may not follow the rules of the church, which when broken send them to hell. The church thus loses power to control behavior as people wake up to the fact that death is simply part of the life cycle.

But for all of their power as catalysts of social change, the sub-stances are still operating or "manifesting" within individual psyches. When Marcuse speaks of the dissolution of the ego shaped by the established society, he points to something profound about our unnecessary fear of death. While we have begun to understand cer-tain mechanisms at play, we know that these medicines transcend an embodied insight beyond reason alone.

A comprehensive theory of how psychedelics manifest their effects remains beyond the scope of any single work. For those seeking a deeper understanding of the physiology and psychology involved, I highly rec-ommend Jahan Khamsehzadeh's previously mentioned 2022 book, *The Psilocybin Connection*.

What I can examine here in more depth, given my background as a clinical psychologist, are the symptoms and distress psychedelics seem to alleviate.

CHAPTER 5

Understanding and Treating End-of-Life Distress

When discussing psychedelic-assisted psychotherapy for patients nearing the end of life, we are primarily dealing with multiple distinct but overlapping forms of distress—namely anxiety, depression, and physical pain. Anxiety manifests as an uncomfortable vibrational feeling, often experienced in the chest and stomach, which brings with it a sense of imminent doom—like something awful is going to happen soon. The physical vibration of anxiety, though energizing, is predominantly unpleasant.

Depression, on the other hand, is a persistent state of sadness, despair, and loss of interest. Depression entails a pessimistic outlook on life, with the glass being perceived as half empty—or worse, where a blue sky appears gray.

When experienced together, anxiety and depression can make for a deadly combination—fueling one another and often leading to suicidal ideation.

While each of the forms of distress are linked, we can benefit from precision in speaking about them individually as well.

Anxiety

In my research for this book, I heard five common fears surrounding death voiced most often:

1. Fear of Uncertainty: Not knowing what dying may entail or what, if anything, follows.

2. Fear of Hell: An existential terror, inverting the hope and comfort of the notion of heaven into a fear of eternal punishment.

3. Fear of Nothingness: That death is the absolute end of self and consciousness.

4. Fear of Losing Control and Suffering in Dying: That the dying process will involve unbearable pain, loss of control, or capacity. We wish for life to end peacefully when the time has come.

5. Fear of Aloneness or Separation: Being isolated in death or the sorrow of leaving loved ones behind.

The first step to disempowering our fears is to give voice to them. Instead of conducting a detailed inventory of these fears upfront, we will examine each of these fears in more depth at different points throughout the remainder of the book and explore how psychedelics might diminish the intensity of each of these fears. However, to understand how psychedelics alleviate fear and anxiety in the general sense, it helps to establish some clear definitions that I have also found essential in my clinical practice.

At the foundation of the fear of death we find the anticipation of a threat—a clear and present danger.

Death represents the ultimate threat as it implies the loss of self and everything known. Wouldn't emotions of distress, anxiety, and depression, therefore seem rational?

As a clinical psychologist, I distinguish between fears—which can be rational and even vital responses to real situations that call for our attention—and anxiety—which we create ourselves even in the safest of circumstances. Fear senses real danger; it can spur action and help us by guiding us toward the right course of action. For example, if you live on the coast and hear a tsunami warning on the radio, you may feel scared, which causes you to flee to safety. Or, if you're fixing a flat tire on a highway, and you are afraid you could get hit by a car, you might light a flare or call for someone to help you.

Anxiety, on the other hand, results from imagined threats or the anticipation of disasters that are not rationally justified. Anxiety arises from within and serves little purpose but to cause emotional distress.

Fear is an important warning emotion of something that is actually outside of ourselves that has the potential to do us harm. The classic example of fear is seeing a bear in the woods, and then deciding whether to fight or run.

Fear can also bring anxiety with it, but they are not synonymous. Anxiety is characterized by an uncomfortable vibration that brings with it a sense of impending doom that you create for yourself. Anxiety can arise anywhere, even in a completely safe bunker with three-foot-thick cement walls, plenty of air, food, water, and a toilet.

So, while some fear around death may be natural and rational, my role as a clinician involves helping patients discern when fear has spiraled into needless anxiety, and is hindering rather than helping them engage in productive actions to alleviate their distress and live gracefully.

I'm interested in how we condition ourselves to create distortions about death that disrupt our lives with worry, fear, and anxiety. After all, we can't change the fact that we will die. But there is value in figuring out how and why we create anxiety about dying, so we can address it gracefully.

I encourage my patients to view their anxieties as teachers rather than tyrants, asking, "What wisdom have you come to offer? What would you have me see?"

We can all relate to the experience of hearing ourselves by speaking, and saying something out loud that we don't really believe.

We say, "Well, wait a minute, excuse me. I just said something that I don't agree with at all."

That's referred to as witnessing. We're listening to what we're saying while we're saying it and if we don't agree with it, we have the opportunity to retract it.

Psychedelics are helpful tools in this witnessing process for they allow us to dissociate our feelings from our thoughts and allow us to stand back and witness both. Practicing witnessing with psychedelics can lead to applying witnessing techniques in daily life without the need for psychedelics. Like diaphragmatic breathing, I believe witnessing is another essential tool for graceful living.

When we witness anxiety, we feel and see the uncomfortable feelings in the chest and stomach. The most effective way to alleviate these feelings is to engage in slow and steady abdominal breathing. Becoming skilled at abdominal breathing is essential for conquering anxiety without the use of body-numbing medications.

When we are able to discuss anxiety about death openly, the honest conversation around death bridges our sense of separation from one another and helps us appreciate each moment as the gift it is.

Demoralization

Witnessing myself from within during my psychedelic experiences has been an important tool for eliminating my anxiety about death and dying, even in the face of two terminal diagnoses. Nonetheless, for many individuals with a terminal diagnosis, initial anxiety commonly gives rise to a secondary phenomenon: feelings of hopelessness or "demoralization," as it is referred to in a clinical setting.

As Bossis explains, "Demoralization is an awful experience that entails an existential loss of meaning, a sense of personal burden, a loss of hope, and a lack of capacity for meaning making."

While depression and demoralization syndrome share some similarities, such as feelings of hopelessness and loss of meaning, there are important distinctions between the two. Depression is a mental health disorder characterized by persistent feelings of sadness, worthlessness, fatigue, and lack of interest or pleasure in activities. It can have various causes, including genetic, biological, and environmental factors. In contrast, demoralization syndrome specifically arises from a life circumstance, such as a terminal diagnosis, that can make despair seem a logical response.

Another key difference is that while depression often responds to medication and psychotherapy, demoralization syndrome resists treatment with medication, given its situational nature. This resistance to treatment can lead the affected to be diagnosed as "treatment resistant," unfairly blaming the patient for an illness we simply do not yet know how to heal. Treatment-resistant depression and demoralization is a way of blaming the patient by implying that since doctors and medicine cannot heal them, they're "resisting" getting better.

In the throes of despair, one often feels powerless and alone. The notion anyone would choose such anguish is absurd. Our task is not to judge but seek to understand, and find ways through compassion to relieve human suffering in all its forms.

While traditional medications have proven ineffective at treating demoralization, Bossis highlights the transformative potential of what he calls "meaning-making experience."

According to him, psychedelic therapy challenges patients' assumptions about life, death, and the self.

Bossis notes that insights gained during the relatively short psychedelic experience help relieve the despair of anticipating an end—the point at which "whatever myself is stops."

Early studies into psilocybin focused on those with intractable depression because regulators favor approval of drugs for which no treatment exists. Preliminary results suggested that when administered responsibly and paired with therapy, psilocybin helps patients process the emotional, psychological, and existential ramifications of facing death.

Dr. Brian Anderson at UCSF explains the results of his recent study on the use of psychedelics for patients with terminal HIV. He told me:

> In a pilot study conducted by our team at UCSF in 2018 and 2019, later published in *Clinical Medicine* in 2020, we worked with long-term AIDS survivors who had moderate to severe feelings of hopelessness, helplessness, and loss of meaning or purpose, which you often see in oncology and palliative care.
>
> We worked with gay men over fifty who had been diagnosed with HIV/AIDS before effective treatments. They were given terminal diagnoses—told they had months or a few years to live. Although many survived by getting experimental and standard treatments, many were isolated, having lost partners and friends, and the social supports they once had. Some felt survivor's guilt and complex grief over losing so many in their community over the years. Others had other health issues like chronic pain, viral hepatitis, or cancer. They have complex medical histories and were thinking about aging,

frailty, and death from causes other than HIV/AIDS. Although the study had no blinding or control group, we showed that offering a moderate to high dose of psilocybin in an individual setting was safe and feasible early on.

Demoralization is a particularly challenging form of depression, which has resisted existing treatments. Hence, these studies are promising and deserve well-designed follow-up research.

Physical Pain

A third area where psychedelics show promise is in managing physical pain.

Although pain is inherently a physical symptom, it seems that psychedelics may attenuate it through a psychological mechanism.

Personally, I have found LSD to be helpful in managing my pain resulting from both the traumatic motorcycle injury and issues related to compressed and degenerative discs.

Similar to their effect on anxiety, psychedelics' capacity to alleviate physical suffering comes from their ability to help us observe or witness our pain from a distance rather than simply experience it.

This is how I described this experience during my interview with Gisele Fernandes-Osterhold who was conducting studies on psychedelics to alleviate chronic pain.

Dr. Richard L. Miller: Can I sign up to be a subject for the chronic pain study?

Gisele Fernandes-Osterhold: Yes, you may.

Dr. Richard L. Miller: I was only half joking. I'm not really joking because I have chronic pain and I know that psychedelics have helped me a lot in my own experiments. Of course, I think the reason they've helped is they get me to see the pain instead of feeling it. So I get distance from the pain, which helps. Sometimes I become the pain, because when there's nothing but pain, then there's no pain because everything is the same. I use that tool successfully at times.

Gisele Fernandes-Osterhold: That's beautiful. The pain itself and your relationship to it can become all-encompassing. You and the pain merge into one. And then there are moments in which you can transcend the pain and witness yourself in pain.

Dr. Richard L. Miller: I find that taking psychedelics helps me use my inner television set to go to the source of the pain. I know exactly where it is, between two nerves that are pinched. I use my mind's inner camera to go to those nerves and try to relieve them. Sometimes I imagine applying cold to cool them down. Other times I try mechanically pulling the vertebrae apart.

Gisele Fernandes-Osterhold: Yeah. If you were having your session in a facilitated way, let's say in a protocol that involves psychotherapy, you would be not only working with that pain the way you are already by looking at it, studying it, getting in there knowing what helps shift, but then afterward you would take that information and processing and say "Could I do things differently? How do I deal with the pain in my daily life or body? Does the pain lead me to certain thoughts or actions? Do I follow them or not?

There are symbolic and habitual ways in which one engages with pain and the body. Sometimes the pain is trying to slow one down, or is asking for one to do more exercise or to hold the body in a certain way or have certain habits. Sometimes that is something that we listen to, and sometimes that's something we ignore and try to go about it as if we don't know that. It comes back because it's requesting a certain part of us or a certain way of us engaging with our bodies in a way that soothes the pain.

Some of the earliest studies on psilocybin showed benefits for patients with chronic pain. In particular, the work of Dr. Eric Kast revealed that psychedelics seemed to disrupt a cycle that is commonly found in those with chronic pain. This cycle involves not only the struggle with the pain itself, but also the anticipation of future pain based on previous experiences.

Kast found that psychedelics seemed to break that cycle, allowing people to step out of that anticipatory loop and just be in the present moment. "As a result, subjects reported significant reductions in the level of pain and the need for narcotic pain medication," Kast observes.

He first published his research on LSD as a painkiller in 1964. Kast theorized that pain involves both psychological and emotional aspects, including the brain's attentional demands. As LSD disrupts attentional processes and has dissociative qualities, Kast was excited about the prospect that it could be the "ideal analgesic" he had been searching for.

I have found this to be true in my personal experience as well. The psychedelic reduces my anticipation of pain, resulting in a subjective experience of reduced pain. This is because the significant psychological component has been removed, leaving only the physiological aspect of pain.

LIVING IN THE PRESENT

The attenuation of physical pain through psychological means speaks to another way psychedelics alleviate our suffering at the end of life: by allowing us to live more fully in the present moment. During my near-death experience following the motorcycle accident, I credit my survival to being able to stay present to my breathing—a technique I learned at Esalen, as well as from my experiences with psychedelics. As described elsewhere in this book, abdominal breathing is an essential tool for eliminating anxiety by stabilizing the entire system and creating homeostasis.

Microdosing, the practice of taking very small, subperceptual doses of psychedelics, has gained popularity in recent years for its potential mental health benefits and ability to enhance creativity and focus. While the doses are too small to produce the profound alterations in consciousness associated with higher doses, many people report improvements in mood, anxiety, and pain. In my experience, microdosing has been somewhat helpful in reducing my physical pain, but slightly larger doses of about 12–15 micrograms have been even more effective.

When I received my life-threatening diagnoses, I wasn't thrown into a spiral of anxiety and suffering, worrying about a future that may or may not materialize. I had already dealt with fear and anxiety and the whole issue of death enough times over the years that it didn't harsh my mellow. Instead, I just went about my daily life, living every moment in the present.

I would say, "Today I am alive and well. I have food, warm shelter, people I love who love me, and the energy to function." After receiving my life-threatening diagnosis, by staying in the present moment, I maintained my customary lifestyle.

Having the skills to stay in the moment without succumbing to the societally taught anxiety and fear of future death was a matter of practicing the steps that I could take to deal with emotions while going about my daily life.

Of course, it's one thing to tell someone who is dying to "live in the moment," but quite another to get them to experience the present as an unfolding and never-ending gift. Living in the moment takes practice over time.

Both psychedelics and near-death experiences can cause a radical awakening to the present, such that whatever pains or worries we have about the future can recede into the background.

Psychedelics are not a magic pill that suddenly removes all pain, fear, and suffering. Instead, they work by helping patients to witness and reframe their suffering and make peace with life on life's terms.

Even some scientists who have made a career out of studying the effects of psychedelics have resorted to the language of mysticism—not science—to explain the ultimate causes of psychedelic healing. Some have been critical of such nonscience and others more accepting. Bossis shared the following story:

There's a great letter from [Aldous] Huxley to Thomas Merton, the great Christian mystic, where Merton had asked Huxley about psychedelics.

"Why do you promote their use?" Merton asked.

Huxley says to Thomas Merton that despite all the suffering of this world and the difficulties of being a human being, these experiences show us that in the end, it's all going to be alright.

Huxley goes on to say, "It's all love, and it's all God."

That sense that it's going to be okay has always been very striking.

Hopefully in a number of years there will be places people can go to at the end of life in preparation for death and have a session with safe protocol for the psychedelics they use. That's the hope.

In my own case, I continue self-experiments with psychedelics in search of remnants of fear, to heal unhealed wounds, to see through new eyes, and to experience new worlds. In short, to expand my consciousness.

PART TWO

THE STEPS TO DYING GRACEFULLY

With the context established and the mechanisms of action explored, let us now turn our attention to the practical steps one might take to access psychedelic-assisted psychotherapy safely and legally at the end of life.

Let us be clear: this book does not endorse illegal activity. Instead, it aims to provide information to empower readers' choices. Research has demonstrated these treatments' credibility and efficacy when administered appropriately. We will now explore implementing them responsibly, maximizing their benefits while minimizing the risk.

The following pages provide advice accrued through decades of experience, as well as through my conversations with researchers, psychotherapists, philosophers, spiritual guides, and end-of-life caregivers.

The steps outlined include: discerning if the path of psychedelic exploration is right for you, navigating legal landscapes, selecting a guide and therapeutic approach, preparing set and setting, optimizing the experience, integrating insights afterward, confronting your mortality, facing the fear of dying, living more fully in the time remaining, and finally, easing the transition itself.

This guidance is not exhaustive but rather highlights key considerations for those who feel called to psychedelic therapy to address end-of-life distress. With compassionate presence and thoughtful integration, these treatments can provide comfort, meaning, and courage as one's journey culminates.

The journey involves mindful intention, cautious sourcing, proper support, and a profound respect for these potent substances. While the psychedelic path may be challenging at times, it can guide individuals through suffering to acceptance, from anxiety to equanimity, and from fear of the unknown to faith in the eternal.

If one approaches psychedelics respectfully and mindfully, they offer unparalleled potential for healing during one of life's most precious and precarious transitions. Please use this knowledge responsibly and with compassion for yourself and others. Our hope is that these steps will ease suffering and cast light on the passage to the beyond for both yourself and your loved ones.

Confronting Death

During my early experiences with psychedelics, my fear of death evaporated and was replaced by calm acceptance. I understood on a deep level that death comes for us all and that we can only embrace life fully by living it. This insight struck me in my twenties, during a period of health and vitality, and it has since shaped my view over six decades including very close calls with literal death. Although psychedelics at life's end are the focus of this book, one does not necessarily need to have a brush with death or receive a terminal diagnosis, as I did, in order to explore new perspectives on the end of life and death.

Still, discussing death does not come naturally, even when you no longer fear it. For most of my life, I avoided the conversation of death, not out of fear, but reluctance.

I have not desired to spend the precious time of my life talking about death. It's a given that, like everyone else, I will eventually pass away. Death is a natural part of the developmental process: we are born, we live, and we die. So, what is there to talk about and why use up precious life energy speaking about death?

Though intimately familiar with the experience of ego death through psychedelics and my own near-death experiences, speaking openly with my loved ones about life's end remained unappealing. My wife, Jolee, who worked in hospice for over ten years, is quite interested in talking about death while living with a man who has little interest in talking about the topic.

When she and her friends discuss death, I often retort, "Unless you promise I will be able to talk about life when I am dead, I don't want to talk about death while I am still alive."

It took writing this book and interviewing so many people who work in end-of-life care to get me to turn my attention to a topic I would have rather avoided. I did it because I am fundamentally a clinician and when people are suffering, I want to help, even when it involves certain personal sacrifice. In this case, the sacrifice was to delve into a topic—death—which I don't think is worthy of spending life on. However, spending time helping those who fear death is a worthy endeavor to which I have committed wholeheartedly.

In our culture, death, alongside topics like sex, money, religion, and politics, is considered taboo. These subjects are often shrouded in silence, avoided due to fear of embarrassment or conflict. While discussing politics, our personal finances, sex lives, and religion can also be challenging, death arguably remains the most challenging topic of all. Growing up in the 1950s, illness and dying were hidden away from the public eye. People with cancer were ostracized and were talked about behind their backs. During that time, people were afraid to talk about their own cancer, or that of others—almost as if talking about it would increase the chances of getting it. Although we have overcome some taboos, death still remains veiled in mystery for most.

As Gisele Fernandes-Osterhold put it to me:

We must consider the social and cultural aspects of how we handle death because our culture and modern society deny death. It's a death-phobic culture. . . . For a hundred years, death has not only been medicalized but professionalized and unseen.

We deal with the fear of death in ways that avoid it; the fear of death is usually unconscious and repressed. We lack spaces to discuss death, properly process grief, and understand the fear of death.

Paradoxically, she notes:

The further medicine advances to prolong the end of life, the more death is perceived as some kind of ultimate failure. We have so much medicine, technology, and yet you're going to die?

She asks this rhetorically, but the framing makes us think we're somehow doing something wrong by dying. It sounds absurd when we say it out loud, and yet this assumption dominates so much of the subconscious dialogue that never surfaces for long enough to be ridiculed and dispelled.

"It's this paradigm of a heroic condition that everything can be solved with science and we can escape the inescapable," she notes.

Philosopher Charles Bush, who spent a decade working with seniors at the Fort Bragg, California Senior Center, observed a similar avoidance talking about the topic of death in the cafeteria where he served three hundred lunches daily for all those years.

As Bush explains: "Asking somebody about intimate experiences like whether they've had someone close to them die is like asking, 'Would you share a story of the best sex you ever had?' People might want to share, but they probably won't, unless there's an unusually strong reason."

As we get closer to death, the reasons for discussing it become more apparent. There are several important questions you have to ask yourself before it's too late—leaving your family members guessing your desires regarding your last act and final bow.

As the seniors got closer to the end, Bush observed that those with whom he'd developed close relationships shared more of their thoughts and experiences with him.

"For the most part, they didn't seem too fearful, anxious, or avoidant about death," Bush tells me. "They were pretty clear that death was going to happen and that it was probably going to be okay."

Still, discussing death remains difficult, and vital questions often remain unanswered. How and where do you want to die, and, maybe more importantly, how do you want to live your remaining time? For most, openness and curiosity surrounding death either comes too late or not at all.

For many, the most difficult part of seeking psychedelic-assisted therapy is initiating the conversation. You might be afraid of social sanctions or harsh judgments from those who have been deceived by the government into believing that these medicines are the devil's work and that anyone caught with them should be imprisoned. Even before you get to the topic of end-of-life use of psychedelic medicines, you might resist the idea of talking about death at all.

Perhaps it is time we rethink our cultural habit of keeping certain topics taboo. Consider that now, more than ever, it may be healthy for us to be authentic and transparent about all topics, including the most personal feelings and thoughts about death, religion, personal finance, politics, and even our sex lives. This may sound preposterous or impossible, yet I can testify to the fact that when I have had the privilege of being with people who are authentic and transparent, it created a feeling like no other. Transparency is like swimming in pure oxygen, riding on clouds, bathing naked in a waterfall on a hot day, or living in flow.

While there are cultures that maintain strong rituals that ease the transition for the dying, American society has historically been death-phobic on the personal level. Yet, paradoxically, at the theatrical level, American culture seems to be fascinated with death, as evidenced by the popularity of movies that include or portray death. In what we call "action movies," dead bad guys fall like rain from the sky. In war movies, we see body parts flying around the screen, and in mysteries, we see the dead body naked on the table in the morgue. Sometimes, we even get to see the cadaver cut open. But it's still just a movie, and we don't relate to the cold, naked body as our mother, father, sister, brother, son, or daughter . . . yet it could be, and at some time, it will be.

Thankfully, there are efforts underway to shift the conversation about death from a morbid focus on death as the endpoint toward a celebration of life and the unfolding of a life-long process.

YOU'RE NEVER TOO YOUNG TO START THE CONVERSATION

I've often wondered why it's so difficult to have a conversation around death, even as taboo topics had become second nature to me early in my career as a clinical psychologist. What makes articulating thoughts around death so difficult?

Psychedelics have helped me appreciate that language is an accumulation of grunts emoted over thousands of years. Different groups in different areas of the world have developed their own unique form of grunting, which eventually became the languages we know today. These languages, or lyrics, continue to grow and evolve. In addition to the lyrics, the delivery of language through tone of voice, amplitude of sound, speed of presentation, facial expressions, and body language are integral parts of communication. Communication, through lyrics and music, is an energy exchange that we decode. We take in the lyrics and music, ascribe meaning to them, and then choose either to react or respond. Typically, reactions are more impulsive and less controlled, while responses are more reflective and thoughtful. When approaching taboo topics in order to shed light on them to make them more acceptable in our society, it is in our best interests to be responsive rather than reactive.

By adopting a responsive attitude and setting aside preconceptions while using a witnessing approach, we come to realize that there is no inherently taboo communication—it's all just communication.

Psychedelics teach us that the purest form of communication is that of authenticity and transparency. Superficial communication is more like "communication lite." There is still an energy exchange in superficial communication, but it is not as profound as deep communication.

There is a stark difference between a casual comment on the weather and genuinely engaging someone with eye contact and inquiring sincerely about their well-being. Eye contact changes the energy exchange and makes it deeper on an interpersonal level. Have some fun and observe people greeting one another. Notice the eye contact or lack thereof.

Psychedelics in this context can teach us how to decipher communication by understanding the music, the tones, the facial expressions, and the body language.

In June of 2023 I gave a talk at the Psychedelic Science conference in Denver, Colorado during which I asked the audience to turn to the person next to them, look them directly in the eyes, and say, "Hello, my name is _____, and I will endeavor to treat you with dignity, respect, kindness, and love."

Imagine how different the world would be if we all used this greeting instead of shaking hands, which is the ancient way of showing there is no knife or sword.

I endeavor to live my life based on what I have learned from psychedelic experiences. These experiences have taught me that communication is often veiled and complex. Through my experiences, I have learned to peel back layers of complexity and communicate simply and directly. I strive to be responsive rather than reactive, and I will continue to practice deep communication for the rest of my life.

Now back to the end of life, aka death.

Siobhan Greene, president of the Hospice Giving Foundation, advocates for a transformation of language surrounding death, "We don't use 'at the end of life' as our language, we use '*through* the end of life,' because the moment we are born, we begin a trajectory of growth, learning, and development."

She notes, "The end-of-life process begins all through life. . . . If we were able to think about it as the natural process we all go through earlier in life, we would be better equipped as a society to understand it."

When I asked her if families of the dying also avoid the topic, she confirmed my hunch.

"Yes, it's a very difficult topic," she tells me. "People are often afraid to discuss death because of the mystery and taboo surrounding it. However, we believe that by encouraging this conversation, we can shift the focus to the beauty and awesomeness of death, rather than what is scary about it. Essentially, we aim to make people aware of this natural part of life so that they can find joy in it themselves or, at the very least, find peace in it."

There are opportunities at every stage of life to confront our mortality and determine how we want to spend the limited time we have. For those nearing the end, the greatest opportunity is to cherish each moment. And even for the rest of us, confronting our mortality involves a radical embracing of the present—not "killing time" waiting for some future event to happen. Openness to our mortality can happen at any age, and it starts with dialogue.

Catherine Durkin Robinson, our country's first "death doula"—a person providing nonmedical, holistic support to individuals and their families during the dying process—made her mission clear.

"My goal is to normalize conversations about death," she says. "Many people are afraid to discuss it, or perhaps we are discouraged from doing so for various reasons. As part of my job, I help people take a moment, have a conversation, and make it a normal part of everyday life. It's important to invite your family to join the conversation so that we can all be on the same page."

Durkin Robinson explains further, "Those of us who work in this space are confronting our mortality on a daily basis; we tend to live with less fear, and it's because we're around it, we talk about it, we see it, and we know how beautiful it can be."

DOULA FOR A DAY

Although psychedelic experiences helped me come to terms with my mortality decades ago, dealing with the practical details of my eventual demise has been a drag. Dealing with paperwork and logistics seems like a waste of my time. The thought of driving to a lawyer's office to fill out paperwork leaves me thinking of all the other ways I could be spending my time instead. In fact, there are plenty of other things I would rather do than go to a lawyer's office to fill out paperwork.

My wife broached the topic given her experience in hospice, yet I believed accepting the inevitability of dying was enough.

To overcome this reluctance, Durkin Robinson walked me through the questions she explores with clients, acting as my death doula for the day.

My first question was, naturally, "What's a doula?"

Durkin Robinson explained doulas support people through life's transitions, from birth to death. "There are birth doulas, who help people prepare for the very real work that goes into labor and delivery to bring a child into this world. Then, we also have doulas who work with people at the end of life to prepare for the very real work of dying. That's what I do," she said.

The concept intrigued me, making me wonder who typically seeks such services and for what reasons. According to Durkin Robinson, most patients reach out after receiving a terminal diagnosis, with six months to a year left, hoping to shape their remaining time and death on their terms.

Yet, not everyone waits for a terminal condition to start a conversation about their death.

"I have heard from people who have never received a diagnosis or certainly haven't received one yet, and they call me because they want to reduce their fears about death," Durkin Robinson said. "They want to learn about the dying process, because they want to have a different relationship with death than maybe their parents did."

Some of her clients are caretakers of elderly family members, whereas others are "just curious" to live more fully now by confronting mortality's shadows. Durkin Robinson also leads community workshops for people of all ages on "different ways of addressing this fear that so many have about end of life."

This echoed something Siobhan Greene said about death being a process *through* the end of life that can begin at any time during one's lifetime:

> In reality, if we were able to think of death as a natural process that we all go through, earlier in life, we may be better equipped as a society to deepen our understanding. If learning about dying starts in high school or college, there are a couple of major benefits. One is that high school and college students often experience the death of a grandparent, aunt, uncle, or unfortunately, parents or peers. If there's no language for it, if there's no sense of "we have to come together as a community to process this and understand it," it becomes even more difficult and devastating.
>
> Introducing this topic of death at a young age equips people to be prepared for conversation and to understand what grief means. They will know that grief is normal and not something you need to get over.
>
> I think there are so many complexities about dying that if we

don't talk about it as young people we go through our lives, and we miss an opportunity to be there for one another and understand the process.

As both Greene and Durkin Robinson emphasize, confronting death—much like giving birth—benefits greatly from support, regardless of when you begin the process.

"Generally speaking, a doula is there to talk with someone and support them in whatever a good death looks like for them," she explains. "So, we get to know our clients, we talk to them, we find out what their goals are, how they want to live the rest of their lives, and how they want to die, and then we support that journey."

Through conversation, Durkin Robinson helps craft a "good death" for each client individually.

"Over 80 percent of us want to die at home, but over 80 percent of us will die in the hospital," Durkin Robinson notes.

For me, that statistic alone proved reason enough to plan.

"When we have conversations and put a plan in place," she adds, "you increase your odds that you'll have the kind of death you want."

Discussion and planning around end-of-life care provide a degree of control—not necessarily over what happens to us, but how we handle it.

EASING ADVANCE CARE DIRECTIVES

Catherine Durkin Robinson walked me through the basics of advance care planning. I told her that I had made a will but still lacked advance directives stipulating my wishes should I lose decision-making capacity.

"It's putting your plans in place in case certain circumstances happen," she explains, for those who are unfamiliar with the concept of an advanced care directive.

"Do you want to be kept alive by extraordinary measures? Do you want your feeding tube removed under certain circumstances? You need to make sure your family is okay with that and that they're going to abide by your wishes when the time comes."

Advance care planning helps avoid confusion and conflict, ensuring your team knows and can honor your choices. Durkin Robinson's holistic approach transforms the prospect of a daunting and lengthy process of advance care into the possibility of an empowering conversation with loved ones, creating space to express care by ensuring your death unfolds as peacefully as possible for all involved.

Durkin Robinson recommends having a professional in the room to mediate these conversations with "the people who are going to be taking care of you or supporting you." Durkin Robinson says that she often helps her clients go through the advance care form step by step so it's not as daunting.

> Not only is that important paperwork to fill out, but it's important to actually tell your loved ones, your support team, your care team, what you want. It's good to write your plan and then make sure that there are copies available.
>
> When you have the plan in place and your loved ones know that they don't have to guess or worry about their part in it, fear and anxiety are reduced for everyone involved.
>
> A dying plan can be a wonderful gift that you give your loved ones, so that they don't have to guess. So many arguments and fights happen in families because they have no idea what their loved one wants and sometimes they're guessing while some folks disagree with other folks. You can wipe all of that out by getting this paperwork done ahead of time.

A doula can play a critical role in this process—what Durkin Robinson calls tender talks—offering guidance through the paperwork and in discussions with family members or friends.

You might wonder why I am spending so much time on these details as the foundational step towards living more fully—without any reference to psychedelics. The reason is that we, as a society, have suppressed these conversations so deeply that even those of us who have had our minds opened by psychedelics still need to be reminded—lest we save such an important step for the end, when some of us will not be in a condition to share our desires with our loved ones.

If you aren't quite ready to fill out a form written in "legalese," you can still take steps towards confronting the practical realities of your death in the form of a card game. Following our interview, Siobhan Greene graciously mailed me a deck of cards called "Go Wish"—a simple card game for sparking conversation about the end of life in a gentle way.*

The thirty-six end-of-life cards each say something like: "to be kept clean," "to have a sense of humor," "to be at peace with God," or "to not be a burden on my children." She explains, "When you play the card game, you sort out what's most important to you and then you talk about it as a group."

She goes on to share, "One year at Thanksgiving, my husband and I and our daughter and son and their partners sat, and we played the game and had this conversation. It had moments where it was typical with my family, a little irreverent, and everybody got a good couple of laughs out of it, and then there were moments where people had a few tears in their eyes. I remember my daughter saying, 'It'll be messy and sometimes that's okay.'"

Once you've opened the door to these kinds of questions, filling the form out will be easy.

FROM DENIAL TO ACCEPTANCE

Transitioning from denial to a state of acceptance when faced with a terminal illness is a profound journey, and psychedelics can play a significant role in facilitating this process. Gisele Fernandes-Osterhold reflected on the process of grief as according to Elisabeth Kübler-Ross, the Swiss-American psychiatrist who served as her mentor early in her career as a hospice nurse. The five stages of grief are denial, anger, bargaining, depression, and acceptance.

"It's been very powerful witnessing people move through those stages," says Fernandes-Osterhold.

---

*You can find the cards on the Coda Alliance's website.

Denial is a danger because it prevents us from progressing to the healing stages of the journey. For those patients participating in her study, Fernandes-Osterhold saw how psychedelics reframe both the internal and external dialogue:

> From avoiding discussing the disease and how it could progress, to facing it, closely examining it, then carrying out life's interactions—whether seeking retirement homes, conversing with loved ones, or realizing "I'm alive and want to live differently now. I have Parkinson's, but that won't limit all of how I live," and everything in that spectrum.
>
> Flipping from thinking in terms of "I will die," to pondering how and when I'll die, and talking to loves ones about that, to seeing how I'm living and making new decisions orienting towards life are all part of the process.

For many people, having heart-opening conversations can alleviate much of the distress surrounding dying. It can also be an opportunity to discuss another great taboo in our culture: the topic of psychedelic medicine. If you are considering seeking treatment with psychedelics, you will want as much support as possible from your family and friends. This begins by telling them about your plans.

Discerning Candidacy for Psychedelic-Assisted Psychotherapy

During the 1980s, I served as director and chief clinician of the Cokenders Alcohol and Drug Program, which I created to address the epidemics of that era. During that time, I witnessed cases of heart failure, respiratory arrest, and psychotic breaks in emergency rooms across the country.

The culprit?

Not LSD, psilocybin, MDMA or ayahuasca.

It was cocaine.

Every drug has what the pharmaceutical industry calls "side effects," a term they use to sanitize and downplay the severity of adverse effects. However, we all know that so-called side effects affect the whole person and they don't just happen "on the side." I call these adverse effects "unwanted complications of medicine" (UCM). Some UCM are present in psychedelics, and advocates for their medicinal potential, including myself, must be fully transparent about these UCMs, rather than acting like pharmaceutical companies who try to conceal them.

If you are considering psychedelic medicines to alleviate end-of-life distress, you deserve transparency and comprehensive information to decide whether you are a candidate for treatment.

It is noteworthy that there haven't been widespread reports of people showing up at emergency rooms with unwanted complications of psychedelic medicines. But anyone considering psychedelic medicines for themselves or others should be informed about the potential unwanted complications and undergo a thorough screening by a competent professional to ensure they are not at serious risk for adverse psychophysical effects.

Scientists Dr. Charles Grob and Roland Griffiths —both vanguards of the renaissance of psychedelic research—have gone to great lengths to establish a baseline of subject safety and make the case for regulatory approval of their clinical research trials and, eventually, for legalization of these medicines.

In the earliest studies by Grob and his colleagues, they excluded patients over a certain age. However, since their initial results showed minimal complications, the latest studies have begun accepting older patients.

As Grob explains, "We are raising the upper age limit. Psychedelic research, for a very long time, was playing it safe and basically excluding subjects over sixty or sixty-five, or perhaps seventy. For modern studies, we're taking all comers as long as they fit the overall criteria. People will not be excluded by age."

When screening patients for recent end-of-life studies, many participants selected for treatment with psychedelic-assisted psychotherapy have been in their seventies and eighties. The only inclusion criteria was for them to have a terminal diagnosis giving them two years or less to live.

Studies on patients with terminal diagnoses inherently involves a group at higher risk. However, age alone is not the most significant factor; rather, it is the presence of other age-related conditions, such as heart disease, that play a role in determining eligibility.

Dr. Grob tells a story about a seventy-four-year-old man, not a patient in his studies, who had decided to try mushrooms for the first time.

"He took a moderate to high dose," Grob relays, "and within an hour, he had expired."

The autopsy report revealed cardiac arrest as the cause of death, illustrating the potential dangers of taking psychedelics outside of a controlled setting.

"He may have had underlying arrhythmias, possibly AFib,* which were triggered by the psilocybin," Grob reports. "This highlights the fact that we have a lot to learn about the effects of psychedelics on cardiac function, especially in people with underlying vulnerabilities, which are more likely to be found in older individuals."

As a pioneer in this new round of research, Grob is a stickler for safety. In fact, all of the researchers I spoke to emphasized how carefully they screen participants to minimize the two broad categories of risk: physical and mental.

Whether you are thinking of enrolling in a clinical trial (see clinicaltrials.gov) or finding an alternative pathway to psychedelic-assisted treatment, there is critical value in taking a meticulous approach to screening.

PHYSICAL CONSIDERATIONS

Some of you may know that psychedelic chemist Alexander Shulgin and his wife Ann Shulgin lived well into their ninth decade, experimenting with novel mind-altering compounds for their entire lives without any apparent or lasting negative effects. Albert Hofmann lived to be over one hundred, regularly using LSD—the chemical he first synthesized while working at Sandoz Laboratories. While it is unknown whether psychedelics can increase lifespan, they can provide a greater sense of meaning to life—which may well be one of the major contributors to increased longevity.

As individuals age, their health risks increase for all kinds of activities, and psychedelics are no exception. According to psychedelic researcher, author, and psychiatrist Dr. Julie Holland, having a psychedelic

---

*Atrial fibrillation (AFib), is a heart arrhythmia—or irregular heartbeat—that can cause symptoms such as shortness of breath, fatigue, chest pain, and dizziness, as well as life-threatening blood clots. AFib occurs when the heart's upper chambers (atria) beat irregularly and out of sync with the lower chambers (ventricles). Most often AFib corrects itself within a few days. Abdominal breathing and meditation can speed up the recovery process. Sometimes AFib can become persistent in which case medications and even medical procedures, such as cardioversion or even ablation, are required.

experience is generally safe as long as there are no significant complicating medical factors. As a good proxy, if the person is able to tolerate moderate to intense exercise, they can probably handle the intensity of the psychedelic experience.

For those with heart conditions or hypertension, psychedelics can pose certain risks.

Clinical psychologist Anthony Bossis points out, "There are some cardiac risks for high-dose psilocybin and other compounds. Psilocybin increases heart rate and blood pressure, so if someone came into the trial with a known cardiovascular history, such as high blood pressure or AFib, that would be an exclusionary criterion."

Dr. Brian Anderson, a UCSF psychiatrist, agrees: "An arrhythmia would be a significant concern. You would think twice about giving someone with AFib a high dose of a psychedelic medicine. Cardiovascular health must always be considered with psychedelic-assisted therapy. Most studies have excluded people with major heart conditions, so there is little scientific evidence to guide the appropriateness of psychedelics for them. Certainly further assessment of risks and benefits is needed."

As Grob tells me: "Classic psychedelics primarily affect the 5-HT_{2A} receptor, but there are other sub-receptors as well, such as 5-HT_{2B}. These receptors are found on heart valves and help maintain their structural and functional integrity. Damage to the valves increases the risk of congestive heart failure and serious arrhythmias."

Having a pacemaker, as I do, presents uncertain risks. Anderson cautions me, "You might be asking for trouble." Since installing the pacemaker/defibrillator three years ago I have continued to self-experiment with LSD and MDMA with no adverse effects, but the risk is there. In my case, at 85, I can be somewhat cavalier for it is certainly too late to say, "he died so young."

Hypertension, or high blood pressure, can be controlled, as can tachycardia—a condition where the heart beats faster than normal, typically above a hundred beats per minute. Tachycardia can be a symptom of various medical conditions or a side effect of certain medications. When using psilocybin, as with any other medication, risk of tachycardia in certain people must be carefully addressed.

Advanced Pain

For individuals experiencing severe physical pain, a psychedelic experience may be too overwhelming or uncomfortable to derive sufficient benefits from to make the experience of enough value. Psychedelics amplify physical sensations which can potentially cause physical pain to become the primary focus of the experience. This shift in focus can make the important psychological inner work very challenging or even impossible.

Bossis tells me, "We've never had to stop a session due to a subject going outside of the parameters we set for heart rate and blood pressure because we're screening out untreated hypertension and heart rate issues. In a healthy person, blood pressure and heart rate are slightly elevated without risk. We've had no serious adverse effects or events."

In Grob's studies, there was no significant increase in blood pressure. In his published work he makes it very clear that "both diastolic and systolic blood pressure need to stay within set parameters providing safety." When asked about it, he explains:

And when there is risk of unsafe elevations, we use a moderate [instead of a high] dose. We didn't have any problem with blood pressure regulation. But you're right, as one ages, one's blood pressure regulation becomes more sensitive.

MDMA appears to come with greater risks than psilocybin for cardiovascular events, given that it contains amphetamine, which has a direct effect on the heart. All of my colleagues who I have asked about this risk have advised caution.

With larger doses of psilocybin and LSD, it is more likely that you will lose the ability to walk or maintain balance. Don Lattin shared with me his experience with ketamine, which has mind-altering dissociative effects—especially at higher doses and when administered intravenously. Lattin recalled an experience in which he self-administered ketamine and fell from the table he was lying on. While he was not injured, this serves as a cautionary tale and reminds us that supervision is essential when administering higher doses of psychedelics.

In summary, those with certain cardiovascular conditions or physical challenges should exercise caution when considering psychedelic-assisted therapy as the experience might be psychologically and physically too taxing.

Physiological Unwanted Complications of Medicine, AKA Adverse Effects

1. Increased Heart rate and Blood Pressure: Psychedelics can cause temporary increases in heart rate and blood pressure, which serve as warning signs for individuals with pre-existing cardiovascular conditions. Some perceive the increased heart rate as anxiety.
2. Dilated Pupils: Many psychedelics cause pupil dilation, which can lead to sensitivity to light.
3. Nausea and Gastrointestinal Discomfort: Some individuals experience stomach discomfort, nausea, or vomiting during the onset or duration of certain psychedelic substances such as psilocybin and ayahuasca.
4. Sweating and Changes in Body Temperature: Psychedelics can cause sweating, fluctuations in body temperature, and feelings of warmth or coldness.
5. Dizziness and Coordination Difficulties: Disturbances in balance and coordination can occur, increasing the risk of accidents or falls.
6. Sleep Disturbances: Psychedelics can disrupt sleep patterns, leading to difficulty falling asleep or experiencing vivid dreams.
7. Headaches: Some individuals experience headaches or migraines during or after the use of psychedelic.

PSYCHOLOGICAL CONSIDERATIONS

Psychosis and schizophrenia are the chief mental health risks, for which clinical studies have carefully screened their subjects.

Many people who lived through the 1960s still have a perception of psychedelics—fueled by government disinformation and media propaganda that substances like LSD cause chromosomal breaks and could turn otherwise mentally-sound individuals insane with just one dose. The jarring fake stories along with tales of people taking LSD and jumping out of windows has misshaped the popular view of psychedelics for half a century.

We now understand that individuals with a personal or family history of psychotic disorders should avoid psychedelics until we have better tools for managing the risks of psychotic episodes possibly being triggered by high doses of these substances. There are no definitive studies in this area as individuals with psychotic conditions are typically excluded from clinical trials, leaving us to rely on anecdotal evidence.

Jahan Khamsehzadeh, author of *The Psilocybin Connection*, believes that psychedelics can potentially be useful to everybody—including those that are suffering from mental health conditions—but our culture and society currently lack the means to facilitate this safely. He says:

> I think we are currently unable to serve people with schizophrenia and borderline personality disorder. One reason is that they can be so ungrounded, and we don't want to give them medication that causes ego dissolution when they might actually need ego strengthening. They might have to deepen their sense of self to find a way to function in this world.

Psychedelics create a holotropic state, a state that naturally moves towards healing. However, some people might need an entire team or clinic that is available 24/7 as their psyche restructures and learns to heal itself. So, I think we will get there. One day, psychedelics will benefit everybody but right now, we do not have the capacity to hold space for everyone.

Special Attention for Those with
Substance Abuse Disorders

In 1985, I attended a seminar at the Esalen Institute in California. I was invited because of my pioneering work with Cokenders Alcohol and Drug Program. The Esalen group asked me about the appropriateness of psychedelics for people dealing with chemical dependence. I said psychedelics could benefit many but also highlighted the risks involved. Some may use the psychedelic medicine as the road back into their addiction under the flag of a drug is a drug. I suggested that psychedelics wouldn't be a responsible treatment modality for this population until we had more insights from research. It's similar to when those who have been clean or sober for a long time think they can start using drugs or alcohol again in a "controlled way." A few might manage it, but since we can't tell who can and who can't, it's risky to say it's okay for everyone. In addition, stopping the use of the drug of choice is only one part of chemical recovery. One must also recover from the chemical dependence lifestyle often involving lying, cheating, and stealing.

For similar reasons, studies commonly exclude those with a risk of self-harm and those showing suicidal ideation. As Khamsehzadeh says, "You have to be willing to feel the entire spectrum of emotions. You have to be willing to walk through hell, because when conducted properly it can lead to a walk through heaven."

Psychedelic experiences can be psychologically challenging and may confront you with difficult emotions or parts of yourself you were previously unwilling to face.

As Khamsehzadeh tells me, "There are risks of trauma or shadow aspects emerging in the experience that one is not yet ready to encounter or integrate."

INTERACTIONS WITH OTHER MEDICATIONS: RISKS OF MIXING SSRIS AND MAOIS

Psychedelics can interact negatively with psychiatric medications.

Andrew Penn informed me that the UCSF study generally required people to discontinue antidepressants before enrolling for psychedelic therapy (Raison et al. 2023).

"The reason for that is twofold," Penn says. "One is that certain antidepressants do seem to attenuate the effects of psilocybin, and the other is around the fidelity of the data."

In other words, it can be difficult to determine the cause and effect of psychedelic medicine when other medications are also involved. While the mechanisms of traditional antidepressants and psychedelics are very different, the potential for one to obscure the effects of the other remains.

Beyond the confounding effects on the data, certain combinations of medications result in what are called contraindications—situations in which a certain line of treatment becomes risky to the patient.

The ethnobotanist Dennis McKenna described one such contraindication of ayahuasca for those taking SSRIs (selective serotonin reuptake inhibitors):

> It [death] is rare, fortunately. Usually, it results from people not observing the right safety protocols. The most important safety protocol to observe is discontinuing SSRI use before taking ayahuasca. Ayahuasca contains monoamine oxidase inhibitors (MAOIs), which potentiate the DMT [dimethyltryptamine] in the ayahuasca. Although MAO inhibitors are clinically obsolete, people frequently take SSRIs, which can interact with the MAOIs and cause serotonin syndrome. This condition can be lethal and is characterized by hyperthermia and other adverse side effects.
>
> The safe protocol is to discontinue SSRIs well before the psychedelic session, usually two or three weeks before, to avoid any potential hazards. Although we often discuss this interaction with due caution, there are no documented cases of anyone dying from this adverse interaction.

An honest assessment of risks and benefits, with guidance from trusted doctors, can help determine if these powerful experiences are right and safe for your unique situation. The opportunity psychedelics provide is too precious to squander, but also too perilous to approach without caution.

We must continue to research the unwanted complications of psychedelic medicines, without worrying that making this information public will cause a backlash or slow progress in the political arena. Psychedelic science is obligated to embrace transparency. To meet this need, I am presently engaged in writing a book titled *Psychedelic Medicine: Adverse Effects,* which will dive deep into this arena.

Franklin Roosevelt's wisdom rings especially true in the realm of psychedelic medicines: "The only thing we have to fear is fear itself."

Navigating the Legal Landscape

In the early 2000s, I went to Israel with a group of scientists led by Rick Doblin, the founder of MAPS, to advocate for the use of MDMA to treat the growing number of citizens suffering from PTSD. The Israelis were experiencing frequent terrorist attacks, with people witnessing horrific scenes in public areas.

During our trip we met many high-ranking government officials including the Chief Justice of the Supreme Court. After one of our meetings the Chief Justice put her arm around me and said, "Richard, we would love to use MDMA with our people suffering from post-traumatic stress disorder. But if we did so, the United States government would sanction us so severely that it would not be worth it, so we can't do it."

This statement underscores the enduring impact of the notorious Harry Anslinger, the first commissioner of the Federal Bureau of Narcotics, which later became the Drug Enforcement Administration (DEA), and former US President Richard Nixon.

Unfortunately, due to Anslinger and Nixon, MDMA was added as a Schedule I controlled substance. The passage of Reagan's Anti-Drug Abuse Act of 1986, which established harsh penalties for psychedelics, further discouraged the progression of psychedelic science.

One of the first signs that the government was approaching rationality came in 2001 when researcher Dr. Francisco Moreno of the University of Arizona obtained approval for a small study with nine patients on the use of psilocybin and obsessive-compulsive disorder (OCD, Moreno et al. 2006). Then, in the mid-2000s, Charles Grob at UCLA and Roland Griffiths of Johns Hopkins established the first psychedelic research programs in decades.

Progress remained slow until the 2010s, when the FDA and DEA approvals for research picked up, and promising results began getting media coverage. The sudden and rapid increase in public interest opened doors for yet more studies.

More recently, respected institutions such as NYU, Yale University, Mount Sinai, and UCSF have joined in exploring the potential benefits of psychedelics for various physical and mental health conditions.

Then, in November 2020, Oregon became the first state to make history by passing Measure 109, legalizing psilocybin, for use in state-regulated services. Voters overwhelmingly approved creating a framework for psilocybin administration in guided, therapeutic settings by licensed facilitators. At the same time, Oakland (in California) and Denver (in Colorado) decriminalized naturally growing psychedelic plants and fungi—allowing individuals to possess them without fear of legal penalty from local law enforcement.

As Andrew Penn, a psychiatric nurse involved in psychedelic research at UCSF, explains: such measures are partly symbolic given the ongoing federal illegality of psychedelics.

However, he adds that these measures also reflect a greater interest in decriminalizing personal use of substances.

"Federal law does have priority over state law in these cases," Penn notes, "but the federal government, since Clinton's time, has chosen not to enforce it."

While promising, local decriminalization alone does not solve the issue of access for those seeking the therapeutic and potentially life-sustaining benefits psychedelics may provide.

An individual diagnosed with a terminal illness may be left wondering what options exist to experience psychedelic therapies legally and safely.

The options for psychedelic therapy are currently still limited to certain states and cities, but state policy changes and approved research studies across the country are starting to open doors. There are also a rapidly growing number of therapeutic retreats available both in the

United States and abroad, often offered through religious organizations that are exempt from federal law.

Until comprehensive federal regulatory approval of psychedelics expands access, those suffering from a terminal illness and seeking psychedelic-assisted psychotherapy are left navigating uncertain legal territory in pursuit of preserving choice and dignity in the relatively little time that remains for them. This is a great injustice in a country founded on the Jeffersonian ideals of personal choice and individual liberty.

In the final chapters, I will explore strategies for organizing and advocating for a legal paradigm shift that balances the historical place these substances rightfully have in medicine, while also acknowledging their potential personal and political risks.

For now, those seeking psychedelic-assisted therapy to grace the developmental path called end-of-life transition have four clear options:

1. Enroll in a psychedelic science study.
2. Travel to a country where psychedelics are legal.
3. Travel to a location in the U.S. where psychedelics are decriminalized.
4. Work with an underground therapist.

As organizations like MAPS work to get psychedelics approved and regulated as medicines federally, I am campaigning to expand local decriminalization efforts across the country. With that said, I cannot condone illegal behavior and must warn the reader that the above options all entail risks—both legal and otherwise.

In the interest of harm reduction, I can provide information to you, the reader, to make the best and most informed decision possible. Let's first look at the "gold standard" option of enrolling in a clinical trial.

ENROLLING IN STUDIES

It seems like only yesterday that I was able to follow every clinical trial in the United States focused on psychedelic medicines. I featured all the leads of the studies on my radio program, and their interviews later became the foundation of my bestselling 2017 book, *Psychedelic Medicine: The Healing Powers of LSD, MDMA, Psilocybin, and Ayahuasca.*

Today, however, such a book would be impossible, as I would need to interview those hundreds of researchers conducting dozens of trials currently taking place on hundreds of subjects with a variety of conditions—from PTSD and mood disorders to alcoholism, and binge eating.

You can find all these studies at clinicaltrials.gov. When you search for the keywords "psilocybin" or "MDMA" along with "end of life," you will see a list of studies that are currently recruiting subjects and those that have been completed.

As of this writing in 2024, the Psychedelic Support Network also provides a clinical trials database that you can search by substance, condition, and location.

These studies will typically provide the best available care in terms of preparation, guidance, and integration for patients before, during, and after the psychedelic experience.

If you are fortunate, you may be one of the few individuals who not only have access to this therapy free of charge but will also be contributing to the advancement of psychedelic research.

PSYCHEDELIC TOURISM

For those able and willing to travel, places like Portugal, Jamaica, and parts of South America offer psychedelic retreats where certain substances are legal or decriminalized. In Portugal, possession of small amounts of all drugs has been decriminalized since 2001, with promising results. Jamaica permits legal retreats offering psilocybin-assisted therapy. For example, Amanda Feilding's Beckley Retreats in Jamaica, run by the Beckley Foundation, is top of the line.

Parts of South America allow ayahuasca ceremonies, as certain indigenous groups have used the brew for centuries.

However, while legal risks decrease in these locations, personal risks may increase without the safeguards present in research or regulated clinical l practice. If you were to experience psychophysical complications while out of our country, you might lack the protections and recourse otherwise available within the U.S.

For those with terminal illnesses, health concerns limit travel options to places where foreign cultures and languages could prove alienating or disorienting.

If you do choose a destination outside of the United States where psychedelics are permitted, it is critical to engage in extensive advance vetting of the retreat centers and facilitators.

In South and Central America, plant medicine retreats are attracting significant tourist dollars—creating something of a psychedelic business boom. Some retreat centers are undoubtedly carrying on a legitimate indigenous tradition, but there are also pretenders, "fly-by-nights," and predators. Given the historical and social context, women can be particularly vulnerable to sexual boundary incursions, especially while under the influence of psychedelics, although all people, regardless of gender, can be particularly vulnerable to breaches of personal boundaries while under the influence of psychedelics.

While certain geographic locations may offer exotic experiences and indigenous cultures, they are not necessarily optimal for health-focused psychedelic-assisted therapy. We need to remind ourselves that psychedelic medicine is a tool within the broader context of personal therapy.

DOMESTIC LOOPHOLES

For those who prefer to stay in familiar settings or are restricted from traveling by health issues, certain legal options for psychedelic experiences exist in the United States. Despite a degree of legal ambiguity, some religious groups have obtained special permission to use psychedelics as sacraments under the First Amendment's guarantee of religious freedom. This grants participants certain legal safeguards when using psychedelics in ritualistic contexts.

As Catherine Durkin Robinson, the end-of-life doula mentioned previously, tells me, "For my fiftieth birthday, I decided I wanted to go to an ayahuasca retreat and I found a beautiful retreat in Orlando,

Florida, where it's completely legal and safe, and it provided just a wonderful awakening for me."

How is this possible given ayahuasca's status as a Schedule I controlled substance? The answer lies in a legal precedent allowing sacramental use of ayahuasca when containing DMT derived from plants, as in this case. Some centers and religious groups that started abroad have established legal branches in the U.S. by partnering with existing churches. The Soul Quest Ayahuasca Church of Mother Earth advertises on its website that it is conveniently located just twenty minutes from Orlando—the tourist capital of the United States. Centers such as these are able to offer what they do because of the Religious Freedom Restoration Act (RFRA) of 1993, which ensures that interests in religious freedom are protected. The precedent was set in 2006 in the case of *Uniao Do Vegetal v. Gonzalez*, and the Supreme Court has upheld this right.

One flaw with this model, especially problematic for end-of-life care, is that churches claiming psychedelics as a sacrament require their members to adhere to a common set of beliefs. In the eyes of the Supreme Court, that's what distinguishes a legitimate religion from a phony religious front group.

Typically, the views espoused by these churches are vague enough that many people can ascribe to them without compromising their own values. However, I believe in the principles of our country's founding that guarantee freedom for *all* religious beliefs—including those who do not possess any religious convictions, or who identify as atheists. So long as proper screening and safety guidelines are in place, psychedelics should be legally available for all adults.

In recent years, the landscape of psychedelic-assisted therapy has evolved significantly. Oregon's Measure 109, which legalized psilocybin therapy, has made progress in establishing the necessary infrastructure. The Oregon Health Authority has been accepting applications for facilitator training programs and is finalizing rules for service centers. The Changa Institute in Portland has graduated over seventy authorized guides.

Colorado has also made strides, with the passage of Proposition 122 in November 2022, which legalized the supervised use of psilocybin and psilocin. The state is currently working on developing a regulatory framework for licensed healing centers. Denver, which decriminalized psilocybin in 2019, has seen a growing number of people seeking out psychedelic experiences for personal growth and healing.

In Oakland, where psychedelics were decriminalized in 2019, community-based organizations have reported positive outcomes for individuals seeking psychedelic-assisted therapy.

Heather A. Lee, a certified psychedelic coach who currently offers her psychedelic retreats in legal settings abroad, explains the complex situation to me as follows:

"In Colorado and Oregon it's legalized, but they haven't fully integrated the infrastructure yet for who can facilitate," she says. "Does it need to be through a center? Who gets the verification and designation as being a center? All of those logistics are still in the works. So, it's a little funky gray area."

Until regulations are established, some skilled practitioners operate in this "gray area" to provide services for those in need, accepting a certain level of legal risk, or partnering with religious groups to overcome federal illegality.

"These decriminalization laws are really saying to the local municipality—or, in the case of Oregon, the whole state—that we're going to disregard the federal statutes on this," says Andrew Penn. "It's similar to how cannabis rolled out almost thirty years ago."

As former Johns Hopkins researcher Katherine MacLean notes, "For psilocybin, I would recommend looking for legal options in the U.S., like the psilocybin centers opening in places like Oakland, Denver, and Oregon. . . . They have licensed therapists and a legal structure set up to provide the treatment."

Lacking enforcement means decriminalization provides some protections for personal use or possession. However, sales, licensing facilitators, and other regulations remain uncertain without comprehensive policy frameworks.

"The best approach is to evaluate underground guides and retreats carefully," MacLean tells me.

UNDERGROUND THERAPY

Of course, the letter of the law does not always have the last word. Prohibition has attempted to stamp out illegal use of psychedelic medicines, but wherever you have a strong enough demand, there will always be black and gray markets ready to meet that demand.

In the next chapter, I will speak more about the risks of obtaining underground psychedelic therapy guides, various therapy types, and dosing considerations. The key factor here is trust.

Taking psychedelics, especially at the end of life or in any vulnerable state, requires an abundance of caution. It's important to vet the guide, the set and setting, the substance of choice, the type of therapy, and the chosen dose. When operating in the shadows of the law, you rely almost exclusively on the trust and reputation of your guide. Recent incidents of abuse that have been brought to the public eye, even by high-profile guides and facilitators, including those who train others to become psychedelic therapists, have taught us that we must be vigilant for the rare predators in our midst.

As policies around psychedelics begin to relax, there are more and better options for legal psychedelic-assisted therapy. However, accessing these compounds safely and legally remains a challenge.

You can improve your chances of safe and meaningful access by thoroughly vetting groups and practitioners, optimizing set and setting, starting slowly with screening for risk factors and using lower dosages, and choosing services that are transparent about their practices and safety measures. We will take up each of these topics in the chapters ahead.

Selecting the Guide, Dose, and Therapy Type

Charles Bush is an eighty-two year-old philosopher and educator with extensive experience exploring his inner depths with psychedelics. A few years ago, when interviewing distinguished elders for my 2022 book *Psychedelic Wisdom: The Astonishing Rewards of Mind-Altering Substances*, I asked Bush about the most difficult experience he ever had with psychedelics.

"I was in a big house with a central staircase that went up and wound around," he recounts, going into his famous storytelling mode. "There was a string hanging down from a light that was up two stories at the top of this stairway."

Cue the suspense soundtrack.

"I came down the stairs, reached up, and pulled the cord. There was a fireplace going in the next room, but the house was suddenly dark. I freaked out. Every aspect of my childhood—[especially] fear of the dark—became completely focused as terror in that moment, and an inability to reach up and grab the cord or tell anybody what was going on [followed]. I was speechless—utterly terrified. I managed to make my way back into the living room where the fireplace was. I got as close as I could to the fire to get its warmth and the glow and just trembled."

You never know what is going to surface during a psychedelic experience. Bush, alone in a dark house, came face to face with his deepest childhood fears. Even though he was experienced with psychedelics at the time, he was not prepared for the unexpected fear he encountered when he found himself alone in the pitch-black house.

Such are the perils of journeying alone.

Finding a trustworthy and skilled guide is the first prerequisite for having a safe and productive psychedelic experience. With the right guidance, fear can be an opportunity for healing. Fear signals our attention, and with proper guidance, we can witness this emotion with curiosity and detachment. Without proper guidance fear can feel overwhelming.

A guide can make the crucial difference between getting stuck in a loop of fear lodged inside of us versus being able to work through that fear and come out of the experience with an attitude of renewed peace, resilience, and confidence in facing one's fears, including the fear of death. However, as we saw in the previous chapter, the illegality of psychedelics makes finding a qualified guide a challenge.

MY OWN TRAINING AS A GUIDE

During the early 1980s, when MDMA was still legal and available to therapists, I was trained by the late Dr. Robert Kantor to practice psychedelic-assisted therapy using MDMA. Kantor was one of the founders and the first president of the Pacific Graduate School of Psychology (now Palo Alto University). He administered 135mg of MDMA at 9:00 a.m. and we began our therapy session. We ended promptly at noon, and I then drove an hour back to my office at the Cokenders Alcohol and Drug Program, in Emeryville, where I resumed consulting with patients by 3:00 p.m.

These training and treatment sessions continued until 1985, when the political establishment, convinced that they had the right to dictate what topics scientists researched, used the draconian tactic of making possession of MDMA illegal. This move was a bold assertion of telling citizens what they can and cannot ingest in the privacy of their own homes. This 1985 ruling by our government significantly reduced the use of MDMA by therapists across the United States, thereby depriving them of a powerful therapeutic tool especially useful in couples therapy. MDMA had already been documented for its ability to reduce defensiveness arising in conflicts, foster vulnerability, and increase empathy.

As a practicing psychologist with decades of clinical experience, I knew within hours of my first engagement with MDMA that it had huge potential for treating a variety of challenging human conditions. These range from discord between life partners and business associates to animosity between political enemies and even warring parties. I came to this deep belief based on the two most prominent effects of MDMA: increased empathy and decreased defensiveness.

Around the same time, I was also trained in psychedelic-assisted therapy with LSD, psilocybin, and ibogaine by Leo Zeff. He was known as "The Secret Chief," due to his influential yet discreet role in the early application of psychedelic-assisted therapy, always working under the radar to avoid legal scrutiny. Despite his passing in 1988, Zeff is still regarded as one of the world's most famous psychedelic guides. During the 80s, Zeff and I lived on the same block in Kensington, California. He would walk down the street with his magnificent smile, come into my living room, and open up his JICS (Just In Case Stash). Zeff would proceed to take out the earphones, eye shades, and a small vial of LSD containing the lesson for the day. During the session, Leo was a master at doing as little as possible. He always chose classical music, but over time, I declined the music because during one long Beethoven session, I became so obsessed with the composer's genius that I was distracted from the adventure of my own inner landscape. I now prefer silence during these inner explorations and would like to take LSD in an anechoic chamber someday.

I value active engagement in therapy sessions, which is achieved by low-dose psycholytic talking therapy. In high-dose psychedelic therapy, the therapist's role is mostly passive. He or she is there to provide a sense of safety and to act as an insurance policy without imposing or interfering. The therapist in high-dose psychedelic therapy is also there to assist in case of what is called a "bad trip."

A "bad trip" is more of an opportunity to look beyond the persona and address inner demons. This is where the experience, skill, and wisdom of the therapist comes into play. With either low-dose psycholytic therapy or high-dose psychedelic therapy, I recommend the presence of a competent guide to purposefully explore the darker aspects of the psyche and overcome inner fears and threats.

HOW TO FIND A QUALIFIED GUIDE

An ever-increasing number of people are being trained and certified to conduct psychedelic-assisted psychotherapy, but the landscape remains fraught with legal peril, making the traditional methods of credentialing difficult.

Those of us who wish to see this psychedelic-assisted therapy made legal and performed in the open must urge caution when it comes to working with guides in the present sub-rosa context.

Not all underground churches, treatment centers, and guides are of equal quality. The same is true of retreats found in exotic locations abroad, where plant medicine retreats are a booming business. Some facilitators are carrying on legitimate indigenous traditions, or following best practices from the new wave of clinical research, but we need also be mindful that it's all too common to hear stories about makeshift shamans who feign impressive credentials that, in reality, are fabricated on the fly.

Katherine MacLean, a neuroscientist who did research at Johns Hopkins with the legendary Roland Griffiths, cautions, "When seeking any treatment, emotions often run high. The same is true here. Bring an advocate to ask questions and provide support."

Although she is not a guide or licensed therapist nor claims to be one, MacLean is one of the most mature and experienced observers of the world of psychedelics. Her book, *Midnight Water: A Psychedelic Memoir,* published in 2023, is a personal psychedelic memoir.

MacLean suggests asking trusted friends for recommendations, conducting interviews with potential guides, and verifying their training and credentials. Unless properly trained, a guide may not be equipped to handle the challenges that may arise during a psychedelic therapy session.

Despite her extensive experience with psychedelics, MacLean's website contains a disclaimer: "Please note that I am not a psychologist, licensed therapist, or medical doctor, and thus cannot provide therapy, counseling, or medical advice."

This is a common refrain amongst many professionals in the current legal environment. It is considered risky to "aid and abet" in any way an activity that remains illegal.

MAPS, the Multidisciplinary Association of Psychedelic Studies, provides a list of mental health support practitioners who are available for psychedelic integration. However, MAPS also explicitly advises against contacting anyone on this list for psychedelics or psychedelic therapy. Their list is strictly intended for the integration services which take place after someone has a psychedelic experience. The Psychedelic Support Network similarly advertises their list of certified therapists but does not promote them as guides for psychedelic experiences.

THE ROLE OF A GUIDE

The primary purpose of a guide is to provide physical and emotional safety and to help individuals work through fears and difficult emotions that may arise during the journey. Fear is a fundamental element that all human beings encounter. As professionals, we cannot stress enough the importance of examining our fears. A guide can make all the difference in having a positive and meaningful experience.

Jahan Khamsehzadeh, creator of the Psilocybin Peer Supporter Certification Program, summarizes the role of a guide as follows: "A guide [is] somebody who has gone through the territory that can bring a deeper sense of safety, can help you explore yourself, and who creates a container for this experience. Fear is mitigated and brought down through a guide, a lot of preparation, or having a lifeline—somebody there just watching you, taking care of you."

While professional guides are ideal, the duration and intensity of psychedelic experiences can make this option prohibitively expensive for many. A professional's time can be expensive, with many hours required for a single trip. A psilocybin trip typically lasts between four and six hours, and up to eight hours with a booster* whereas an LSD trip typically lasts anywhere between eight and twelve hours.

As Khamsehzadeh notes, "The main challenge [. . .] is accessibility, both in terms of cost and availability. However, as we move forward and laws begin to relax, psychedelic therapy will become more accessible."

For those unable to work with a professional guide, other options include training a friend or family member to serve as a guide.

ACTIVE VS. PASSIVE GUIDES

Guides for psychedelic experiences are generally categorized as active or passive. Active guides conduct low-dose psycholytic therapy and passive guides conduct high-dose psychedelic therapy.

Active guides take an engaging role during the experience. They initiate conversations and may provide prompts or questions for exploration. Lower to moderate doses are typically used to allow for open communication.

High doses on the other hand, particularly "heroic" doses of psilocybin or large doses of LSD, make the person much less likely and inclined to communicate. Here, passive guides hold space by being present and supportive, without judgment, allowing the person to express their feelings and thoughts.

Passive guides maintain a safe setting and remain available as a supportive presence should the individual wish to talk or express emotional distress.

For example, if the person asks, "Where do you think I should go next?" a passive guide might give a simple directive to prompt the person to ask themselves about their next direction.

The guide might respond with, "Close your eyes and see what comes up. What kind of topics do you think would be best for you to look at?"

---

*A booster refers to an additional dose of a psychedelic substance, typically taken a few hours after the initial dose, to extend or intensify the experience. In the case of psilocybin, a booster dose may be taken around the two- to three-hour mark to prolong the effects for an additional two to four hours.

A passive guide encourages self-reflection through the use of warm, friendly language and carefully avoids influencing the individual's journey by suggesting what *they* think is interesting or where the person should go.

In the original Johns Hopkins study on terminal cancer patients (Griffiths et al. 2016), guides took a passive role, given the large dose of psilocybin being administered.

As MacLean explains, "We tested a high dose of around 25 to 30 milligrams per 70 kilograms of body weight, which equates to about four to five grams of dried mushrooms."

Terence McKenna, the late psychedelic explorer and brother of renowned ethnobotanist Dennis McKenna, popularized the term "heroic dose" to describe the powerful experience of taking five grams or more of dried mushrooms. At this dose, the patients in the Johns Hopkins study generally experienced medicine lying down—with an eye mask and headphones to facilitate the deep "inner work" of identifying and confronting fears around death and dying.

A high dose of psilocybin still allowed most participants to retain a level of awareness that permitted some discussion and inner work. This is how Griffiths describes the experience when I interviewed him alongside MacLean back in 2013—shortly after their pioneering and groundbreaking results were published:

> People take the capsule and are invited to lie down on the couch, they're encouraged to use eye shades, so they're going inward, and they're using headphones through which they're listening to a program of music—largely classical, some world music. It's a very introverted or inward-turning experience. That's the nature of the experience. We invite them to simply go in and explore, so there's nothing guided about this experience. They have two monitors who are sitting in the room, very often right by their couch. They are there to provide support, and a reminder of what consensual reality might be like, should they lose bearing of that at the high dose of psilocybin that we administer. . . . Under these conditions, psilocybin produces all kinds of alterations and perceptual phenomena:

visual, auditory, and tactile. It produces marked changes in mood and affect, and thought processes.

The dramatically intensified experience of a high dose, as MacLean notes, may lead some into a state of "cosmic consciousness," where the usual sense of self or the awareness of surroundings fades away. While such experiences can be profound, they may not produce lasting insights or benefits after its effects have subsided.

The impact of psychedelics greatly depends on the dosage, which should be carefully considered to balance the intensity of the effects with one's capacity to process and integrate them.

ENTERING MYSTICAL CONSCIOUSNESS: WHAT IS A HIGH DOSE OF MUSHROOMS?

When I first spoke with MacLean, she was working with Griffiths at Johns Hopkins. In our second interview, a decade later, we revisited the academic work she left behind and she reflected on the employed protocols. On the topic of what constitutes a high dose in their research, she comments:

> At Hopkins, we were mostly studying psilocybin,* which is one of the main chemicals in magic mushrooms. We tested a high dose of around 25 to 30 milligrams per 70 kilograms, which means in terms of dried magic mushrooms, for anyone out there who knows this, it's about four to five grams.

Our conversation shifted to LSD. There's a certain number of micrograms of LSD which creates a significant change in consciousness but one is still able to both converse and do inner work, such as working on the ego and possibly even experiencing ego death. There's a micro-

---

*It is important to note here that there are two distinct types of psilocybin. One type is the psychedelic mushrooms which are measured in grams and the other is the laboratory-created psilocybin measured in milligrams. The laboratory created psychedelic is much more accurately administered as mushrooms can vary in intensity.

gram dose of LSD above which you go right past the ego level and into cosmic consciousness. MacLean explains:

> I would say that we were right on the precipice of that boundary at Hopkins. Some people were able to stay aware of the room, the guides in the room, their body, their own biography, and dip their toes into cosmic consciousness. Some people went a little bit over that edge depending on their body weight and experience. Most people had never tried a psychedelic before our studies, and some people went straight into cosmic consciousness.
>
> The lovely thing about their journey is that they were in a really safe place. With two guides in the room, music, a lovely setting, and no way to hurt themselves, it was a completely safe and potentially awesome experience to have. Of course, not everyone loved it, but for the most part, we were kind of balancing that space between awareness of consensus reality and what you call cosmic consciousness. We called it mystical consciousness at Hopkins.

In my experience, I find that the most productive mental state is just below cosmic consciousness or mystical consciousness. This is where I can initiate changes in my behavior, communication style, personal fears, and creativity. If I am working on a project during this state, I can take notes or record my thoughts for later use.

While cosmic consciousness is a wonderful experience, I often find that I don't have many takeaways other than the experience itself. It's like a ride at Coney Island—exciting, but not very useful in everyday life. When I ask MacLean whether her research found these two mental states to be distinct, she replies:

> I can relate to it. The potentially fascinating thing that we found is in the way we prepared people, we used psychedelic pioneer Bill Richards's mantra: trust, let go, be open. People have the freedom to fully surrender to that greater experience—the beyond, above, under.

What we suggested is that people try not to take notes or remember anything, and then at the end, they would tell us everything they could remember. Through writing, discussions with us, and many scientific measures, we could determine what was remembered—perhaps unconsciously or subconsciously—that might be normally lost to a recreational drug user.

In subsequent chapters, we will turn to the topic of psychedelic integration, but not before concluding the choice of dose, which depends on the kinds of guides you have access to, as well as the mode of therapy that you feel is most conducive to your healing process.

CHOOSING A DOSE:
START LOW AND GO SLOW

One question that often arises from those without prior experience is, "How do I know how much to take?"

Some may feel called to jump headlong into Terence McKenna's "heroic dose" in silent darkness. While this may induce a profound mystical experience, the intensity of effects also increases the possibility of psychological trauma without proper preparation and guidance.

As Khamsehzadeh cautions, "What I have seen in a few people is that it can be traumatic, because you can buy into this idea of [ego] death, and your body doesn't know the difference. That trauma can stay with you for a while."

Recall the quote on the door above the monastery at Mount Athos: "If you die before you die, then you won't die when you die."

Ego death can be educational, beneficial and spiritually profound. The question is how to get there with the most grace and the least unnecessary trauma.

As Khamsehzadeh notes, "If somebody's there and telling you that you are safe, instead of five hours in that trauma state, you can overcome it in five minutes.

For solo explorers or those without access to professional guidance, building familiarity through a gradual approach undoubtedly remains the safest path.

For those new to psychedelic experiences, the adage "start low and go slow" applies. Microdoses such as 0.1 grams of mushrooms or low to moderate doses such as 1–3 grams of mushrooms allow one to build familiarity with the effects before moving to higher doses. Khamsehzadeh advises: "Historically, indigenous people have believed that you are building a lifelong relationship with plant teachers. . . . Probably the safest and easiest route is microdosing. . . . It could help your system build a tune with this compound and get used to the subtleties of the altered state. There's enormous benefits, including alleviating depression and anxiety."

LEARNING TO ILLUMINATE THE DARK PLACES WITH HELP

Charles Bush's re-living of his childhood fear of the dark did not end with him trembling until the effects of the psychedelic wore off. Instead, his wife found him curled up in front of the fireplace, embraced him, and rocked him as he silently recovered his senses.

After some time had passed, Bush was able to express what had happened as his wife comforted him.

"You got afraid of the dark. Everything's okay. Nothing terrible is happening. This is coming from the inside," she said.

As Bush began to relax, they walked back into the hallway and looked past the spiraling staircase to the original source of his terror.

"I began remembering being in bed [as a child] and being terrified," Charles recalled. "I began to understand that it was a whole lot of complex things connected with my early experiences of the dark and wanting mommy and daddy. I was able to experience pure terror, and then see that the pure terror was not connected with anything frightening. I not only got to experience probably the deepest fear I've ever had, I also got the fear to unravel and got to feel its roots in childhood terror. None of it had actually hurt me."

While profound or mystical experiences catalyzed by high doses of psychedelics can be meaningful when prepared and guided properly, they can also be overwhelming if you are unprepared or when you are attempting to process your fears alone. Thankfully, Bush was not alone that night in the big house. He had a guide who was there at the right moment to prevent his experience from turning into one of hours-long terror.

Integrating insights gleaned from any state of altered consciousness is a long process, in which the right guidance is crucial.

In the following sections, we will explore strategies for maximizing the insights and value derived from psychedelic experiences and how to incorporate them into everyday life.

STEP 5

Managing Set and Setting

About an hour into my first psychedelic experience after swallowing four hundred heavenly blue morning glory seeds, a loud, persistent banging invaded my awareness. My mind seized on a story: we were in trouble for taking LSD, and the noise signaled authorities coming to end my career before it began. I was terrified, until I opened my eyes to find its source. There, outside the window, telephone linemen were hammering at their task installing wire. I laughed until I almost cried.

My frightful fantasy, conjured in a moment of vulnerability, revealed how profoundly external factors can impact one's experience. The narratives we construct in our minds have power. Set and setting are not addendums but imperatives to navigate psychedelic space effectively.

Researchers have extensively discussed the influential factors of "set and setting." The "set" (mental state) and "setting" (physical environment) can make all the difference between a transcendent healing journey and a temporary nightmare such as I had during my first psychedelic experience. While I believe that a "bad trip" has the potential to bring to light important insights, such as fears to be processed, we certainly want to carefully avoid introducing any unnecessary complicating factors such as loud sounds, machine-made physical vibrations, voices, unrelated music, and similar distractions.

As psychedelic pioneers in the 1960s and 1970s came to realize, environmental conditions profoundly shape the experiences that unfold.

Later, in the 1980s, a similar recognition of environmental factors came to light with the discovery of MDMA by recreational users, who, enthralled by its heart-opening properties, attended raves while on the drug without knowing the importance of hydration, body temperature regulation, emotional toll during "comedown period," and cardiovascular contraindications such as AFib. How easy it was for the culture to forget that the "A" in MDMA stands for Amphetamine.

From these important historical lessons we have learned that a carefully curated special setting is a major contributing variable toward productive psychedelic therapy.

Acknowledging that a comfortable and disruption-free environment is essential for psychedelic-assisted therapy, clinical studies such as those at UCLA and Johns Hopkins had to go to great lengths to transform the rooms in approved medical facilities into aesthetic living-room-like environments that felt warm and cozy rather than cold and sterile.

The room in which I'm writing right now would be an excellent setting for a psychedelic journey because it offers indoor shelter with views of nature through glass walls. Such environments, akin to prescription-grade nature (RxN), are often deemed perfect for psychedelic therapy.

For lower doses in self-directed or conversational psycholytic therapy, outdoor settings can be suitable, weather permitting. The key is to choose a place free from potential interruptions. For lower doses you might also select a beach that's not too sunny, windy, or cold, as long as there are no people around you.

It is essential to keep the decibel level in the environment as low as possible during the psychedelic experience. Although it allowed me to confront the fear I experienced during my first morning glory experience involving the jackhammers outside, such environmental disturbances cause unnecessary distress, especially for those looking to address the fears related to end-of-life distress.

Setting Checklist

- Ensure a calm, comfortable, and safe environment free from distractions and interruptions.
- Select comfortable furniture such as a couch or stuffed chair.
- Have cozy blankets and wear loose, comfortable clothing.

- Turn off phones, computers, and other electronic devices to minimize distractions.
- Use earplugs or noise-canceling headphones to facilitate introspection.
- Use eye masks to block out light and other visual stimuli.
- Have water and snacks available.
- For guided experiences, choose an experienced and trustworthy guide who can screen you for risk factors and create a controlled, safe and supportive environment.
- For higher doses, consider spending the first half to eighty percent of the time wearing eyeshades and the remainder with the option to take them off.

SET OR MINDSET AND INTENTION SETTING

Psychedelic-assisted therapy can be related to mining your own inner gold mine: delving in, exploring, and pulling out insights to polish and refine in subsequent days and weeks. Psychedelics are not magical cure-alls; the profound experiences they facilitate often require significant processing. If you choose this path of treatment, you must be prepared to spend a significant amount of time integrating the derived insights. We will discuss post-therapy integration at greater length in the next chapters, but the integration journey begins with setting intentions before the experience.

Katherine MacLean told me a story that illustrates the power of intention setting as it relates to a psychedelic experience:

A young man approached me and said, "I'm thinking about having my first mushroom experience."

I replied, "Okay, well, I don't sit for people. I've got two little kids. But I'll help you prepare."

For one year, I worked with this man to figure out why he wanted to take mushrooms.

He made so many changes in his life to clear up the space so that he would be ready to take mushrooms.

Then the year came around, and he said, "You know what? I kind of like what I'm doing with my life. I'm going to wait a little longer and keep preparing."

So I consider that a success story. He may take mushrooms at some point.

We can all benefit from taking time for personal reflection, and to be more intentional about how we live our lives.

In the NYU cancer study (Ross et al. 2016), participants went through a preparation period with not just one but two therapists, who helped them review their life, their intentions for being in the trial, and how their cancer has affected them.

"They talk about their fears, and the anticipated loss of connection with this life," Bossis tells me.

Here, too, we can learn from clinical trials as a "gold standard" in developing best practices.

Likewise, in the Johns Hopkins study (Griffiths et al. 2016), participants prepared for two to three months dependent on the dose of psilocybin.

MacLean describes the model they used at Johns Hopkins to prepare for a high dose of psilocybin: "It was not magically created out of thin air. We prepared people for one to two months before their first experience, and some people didn't receive their high dose until they've been with us for another month, meaning they receive three months of preparation in total."

Three months may sound like a long time, but if you have the luxury of time on your side, it may be worthwhile.

When helping a person prepare for a psychedelic journey, I offer people two options for setting their intention. One is to make a list of topics or past experiences you aim to explore.

I believe that spending time before a session to clarify intentions and potential directions is worthwhile. Writing a list provides focus that may bring up topics you wouldn't have thought of otherwise.

On the other hand, I also think there's a place for embarking on a journey of exploration and experimentation with no agenda whatsoever and seeing what happens.

Hence, the second option I suggest is to just show up and be open to whatever may unfold.

If you are unsure what to put on your list of intentions, it's helpful to spend some time journaling, meditating, and clearing your mind to see what comes into view. Take time to allow the stream of consciousness to arise.

SETTING PHYSICAL INTENTIONS

In addition to clearing your mind, you want to go into the experience with as much physical balance and clarity as possible. Here are some of the areas I recommend paying attention to in the preparation phase:

"Clean"—It is best to allow your whole being to relate to the psychedelic substance, rather than being diverted by physiological issues from food or substances. Ergo, eat light and clean the day before. Some people choose to fast overnight, and that is a personal decision as related to how dietary habits affect mood and energy. Keep a supply of water and snacks at hand, even including sweet ones like fruit, as classic psychedelics can cause a sudden drop in blood sugar. I learned about the drop in blood sugar from the British psychedelic researcher Countess Amanda Feilding during an interview.

Well-rested—I highly recommend getting a full night's sleep before the journey and aiming to start around 10:00 am. The experience itself can be both physically and emotionally draining, and you will want to have as much energy going into it as you possibly can. I do not agree with those who begin psychedelic experiences in the evening, such as most ayahuasca practitioners. Starting a six- to ten-hour journey in the evening leads to fatigue in the middle of the night when we are usually sleeping. Best to be your most rested and strongest when taking psychedelics.

Pain-free—Ideally, avoid psychedelics when you are in acute pain unless you are using the psychedelic experience to explore the sensations of physical pain. I advise people engaging in this exercise to focus on the sensation of pain until becoming one with it, at which point the pain may vanish as it has no reference point for comparison.

Prescription Medication—Ensure that no prescription medication you are taking will interact adversely with psychedelics. For example, MAO inhibitors should be discontinued six weeks before and after ingesting ayahuasca and SSRIs should be stopped at least two weeks before and after taking psilocybin or LSD.

Technology—Make certain all phones and computers are off.

Creating space for psychedelic experiences in this patient and mindful way allows for life-changing gifts to arise that persist long after the experience as you walk the path they illuminate.

STEP 6

Surrendering

Hunt Priest, an Episcopalian minister whose name fittingly reflects his vocation, embarked on his religious path relatively late in life, entering seminary at thirty-seven and being ordained at forty.

Twelve years later, in 2016, Priest was given an irresistible opportunity to participate in a psychedelic research study on religious professionals. Led by veteran psychedelic researcher Bill Richards at Johns Hopkins University, two dozen psychedelically naive religious leaders from diverse faiths were given two powerful doses of psilocybin under supportive conditions. The aim was to assess whether these induced transcendental experiences make the leaders more effective and confident in their work and how it alters their religious thinking.

In this context, *naive* refers to individuals like Priest who had not previously taken psychedelics. Despite living through the 60s and 70s, he had never considered psychedelics as tools for expanding consciousness before.

At fifty-two, Priest had his first psychedelic experience with psilocybin as part of a research study.

"Even ten years ago, I would never have thought I'd be doing what I'm doing right now," he tells me.

Profoundly influenced by this experience, Priest quit his secure position as parish church rector and started Ligare—A Christian Psychedelic Society, serving to help other clergy members find safe, competent guides for their psychedelic experiences.

"This is a privileged place to be—to be able to quit one career and start another," Priest acknowledges, drawing inspiration from the

Franciscan mystic Father Richard Rohr to embark on what he considered the "second act" of his life.

Priest's journey highlights our human capacity for radical change—what Christians call a metanoia.

"I wouldn't have gone to seminary and been ordained if I hadn't had similar experiences without psychedelics," he note. But the experience he had with psychedelic mushrooms gave him a different sense of knowing. Through psychedelics, he discovered again that we can awaken to new realities about ourselves and our world at any point.

"What I learned after that spiritual and religious experience is much of what I've been discussing as a priest, much of what I learned in seminary, as a child, and as a teenager . . . it was real," he says.

"God is real; and healing is spiritual healing—energy transfer. It's all real. And we can't explain it, quantify it, or prove it. I don't need to convince anyone else. The words fail."

His mission with Ligare is sharing the lessons of his transformation and helping others do the same.

LETTING GO, AND LETTING GOD

A few years before taking part in the psychedelic study, Priest had attended a ten-day Vipassana meditation retreat where silence is maintained by all participants. On day five, he experienced a strange feeling in his leg.

"I had an experience of an electrical current in my left thigh, sort of a spiraling current, and I thought, 'Oh my God, I don't know what that is, I don't know why that happened,'" Priest recounts. "But that seemed to be so important to this experience. I was having a very embodied experience, and that seemed connected and important."

When Priest went to the psilocybin session years later, he had trouble getting comfortable at first.

"All of a sudden, I feel the same spiraling electrical current in the same place on my thigh." And then, Priest thought to himself, "I had this experience after five days of that difficult meditation experience, and now I'm having it just an hour and a half into this psychedelic experience."

He recalls trusting the experience from that point forward as something legitimate.

"Something in my mind thought, 'Okay, this is real, and this can be trusted,'" Priest tells me. "I let go. I literally just let go."

As soon as Priest surrendered, the experience intensified. He describes an intense electrical current moving up his spine that got stuck in his throat. Priest says, "A couple of minutes in, I started to feel like, 'Oh my God, something's blocked, and it's going to come out.'"

He thought his Adam's apple might explode.

At this point, Priest's guides laid their hands on him to help move the energy in his body. One guide laid hands on his throat, while the other guide had Priest press his feet into his hands.

"Whatever that was—well, the laying on of hands is what we would say in church—caused that electrical current to go up 1,000 percent," Priest recalls. "And this blockage opened up."

With the release of energy in his throat, Priest began speaking in tongues—something typically associated with Pentecostal traditions, but which was almost unheard of in his own Anglican faith.

"I was speaking in words that I didn't understand, and over the course of the next three or four hours, I had this experience of incredible spiritual connection—this incredible sense of healing and understanding something about what happens when we pray with people and lay hands on them—that transfer of energy," Priest describes.

A HOLY DEATH

Priest sees psychedelics as a means for Christians to overcome their fear of death. "Our core belief is that, whatever happens after we die, death does not have the final say," he says. "This is the story of Good Friday and Easter: even in the face of the most terrible and gruesome death, there is always something new that follows, something beautiful, and a new beginning."

However, the church has not only failed for centuries to help alleviate the fear of dying among its followers but has exacerbated that fear through the portrayal of hell as a place of eternal conscious torment.

"Despite the religion's consistent message that death does not have the final say, many of its followers reach the end of their lives feeling scared, angry, and fighting it until the very end," he notes.

"It's unclear how we got here. Part of it may be due to the myth that we can beat death. Modern medical science can help us prolong life— we can beat it for a while. Most of us don't die in our thirties anymore, but we don't die a peaceful, holy death."

He continues, "We've done a terrible job of preparing people in the culture and in the church for what death really means. Death is as natural as being born, and it's not a failure. It's a natural process, just like the tree I'm looking at right now, which will also die at some point."

According to Hunt Priest, there are rituals that can help individuals begin the dying process, but they are not utilized as much as they could be. Many people wait until the last minute to enter hospice because they believe it means giving up —not realizing that it can be a peaceful and holy way to go. Sadly, most people die without experiencing a peaceful, holy death, and some die completely scared.

"The teaching of the church and their faith has not helped them prepare for that, and it's beyond tragic," Priest says. "It's terror. It's unbelievable."

According to Priest, psychedelic experiences allow a glimpse into realms beyond the physical, affirming the Christian idea that death has no dominion. He hopes to guide others to this radical acceptance and release fear's grip. His psychedelic society Ligare aims to educate Christians and the public about the potential of psychedelics for healing and spiritual growth, while advocating for their safe and legal use for anyone who needs it.

For Christians wary of psychedelics, Ligare provides a familiar framework and according language for encounters with the numinous: "The church is about healing. If not, we should shut our doors."

By rooting psychedelic practice in Christian tradition, Ligare allows the faithful to explore the furthest reaches of human consciousness without leaving their faith behind.

The word *ligare* is Latin for "to bind" or "connect," and makes up the second half of the word *religion*. Priest believes the crisis of modern spirit calls for reconnecting with the sacred in new ways. However, change often comes from within and through guides who walk ahead, lighting the path for others. Priest aims to be one of those guides for Christians—translating between doctrine and the radical openness psychedelics revealed to him.

PSYCHEDELIC REVELATION OF SPIRITUAL TRUTHS

For Priest, psychedelics revealed spiritual truths already familiar to him as a priest, though he never grasped them so viscerally. Amongst others were the centrality of forgiveness, gratitude, and community.

Priest emphasizes that forgiveness is Christianity's moral bedrock. He points to Jesus on the cross, alluding to forgiving those who condemned him to a brutal death. "That's our goal—to be people who, when terrible things happen, can forgive," he says.

Forgiveness to oneself proves equally elusive and imperative. Through psychedelics, Priest found grace to release regret and self-judgment accumulated over years.

Gratitude emerged for Priest as a spiritual discipline with power to transform our view of the world.

A practice of embracing each day with gratitude—despite the sorrows it might bring—opens our eyes to the wonder of existence as a gift. For Christians, gratitude expresses faith in new life even in the face of death.

"Gratitude means waking up every morning and feeling thankful for being alive. If we could all do this, it would change how we see each other and ourselves in the world," he observes.

"Community," Priest says, "makes experiences of God and growth possible by providing a 'container' for transformation. Psychedelics foster connection and empathy, dissolving divisions. For Christians, shared ritual and story shape a sense of the sacred. Ligare aims to build community as an 'access point' for psychedelic practice grounded in faith."

Priest's mission is to share a vision of healing and wholeness through radical openness to God's presence—one that conquers even humanity's oldest fear of death. The story of Christ's passion, death, and resurrection highlights psychedelic themes of surrender, loss of ego, and rebirth into new life.

"The church has done a lot of good and a lot of terrible things," Priest admits.

However, at their heart Christianity and psychedelic practice converge on a truth that "everything's okay, everything's as it should be," he says.

Forgiveness, gratitude, and surrender unite to make real the promise of resurrection, leaving fear behind in the empty tomb.

Through psychedelics, Priest rediscovered the faith he already had. His calling is helping others do the same, that they might behold at last what he has seen—and "be not afraid."

Priest's story illustrates how experience and the right kind of preparation can prime us for psychedelic journeys in unexpected ways. His meditation retreat prior to his psychedelic experience attuned him to recognize and trust the energetic phenomena arising during his psilocybin experience. Without that sensitivity, the throat blockage and subsequent release of energy may have seemed threatening rather than healing.

When it comes to the experience itself of taking a psychedelic—and especially taking a large dose—que será será, whatever will be will be. Attempting to direct or micromanage the experience is likely to create more resistance than anything else. Instead, observation and surrender are key.

"I also would say now that there was a kundalini awakening and my throat chakra was blocked," Priest tells me. "I didn't really have that language seven years ago when that first happened to me."

For him, both the act of surrender and the language around it came naturally—in part because of his theological training, and in part because of the powerful previous meditation experience. His guides' laying on of hands also shows us the power of intimacy and human touch to help move energy during psychedelic experiences.

However, Priest's experience also highlights many of the challenges that can arise for someone who is unprepared, or who is being guided by inexperienced hands.

SURRENDERING AS THE SOLUTION
TO THE FEAR OF NOTHINGNESS

While surrender comes naturally to some, it is a difficult skill to master for most.

Thomas Roberts believes that our deepest fears surrounding death stem from our ego's attachment to control as well as a fixed sense of identity. As he puts it, "Our sense of self doesn't want to relinquish control. We fear death because it signifies 'no more me' or 'I won't control things anymore.'"

To overcome this fear, I have found it helpful to embark on what I call "inner space travel." I search within for fears under the rug of consciousness, lurking in the recesses of my mind—and I confront them directly. Time and again, I have found that beneath surface ego anxieties lies a single, primal fear: the fear of death.

To work through this fear, I practice an exercise I learned through psychedelic experiences. I lie down, close my eyes, breathe, and surrender—allowing myself to "die" for a few minutes. I first encountered the feeling of ego death on a large dose of LSD. Throughout my first ego death, I was confident that I would come back to this place in subsequent trips—even when it felt like I was really dying.

Fighting the psychedelic experience or trying to control it makes you more likely to have a challenging time or what people refer to as "bad trips." Surrendering, on the other hand, allows you to enter a different state of awareness, through which healing takes place.

I now practice this form of "dying" as a regular exercise without taking any substances. So far, I have always returned. One day, I may not come back, but until then, it is a fascinating exercise for clearing fear which I heartily recommend trying.

Journalist and author Don Lattin suggests a variation of my practice to engage in search missions surrounding fear of death.

"One of the things that they advise people if, let's say, you have a vision or hallucination of a monster coming at you, is don't run away from it. Face it [your fears] with curiosity," Lattin says. "Ask, 'What are you trying to teach me? What are you trying to tell me?'"

Looking at fear this way can help make life more graceful whether you are dying or not.

Back in our initial interview, Roland Griffiths shared the following story about his lab's 2016 study on cancer patients:

> Some will have an extraordinary sense of panic that will actually open them up into transcendence. It becomes a doorway through which they reach transcendence. We do have a smaller percentage of people who get caught in the classic "bad trip," where they're in a period of anxiety or dysphoric struggle for most of the session. The important thing about those people is that none of them felt that they had been harmed by that experience.
>
> There were people that would say, "I would never, ever, ever want to have that experience again."
>
> But interestingly, we've never had any of our normal volunteers drop out of the study, even though they had subsequent sessions scheduled, because of a difficult experience.

A relative of mine took psychedelic medicine, and for over five hours he was screaming, yelling, and regurgitating—anxious and panicked throughout the experience.

When I spoke with him later he said, "Sure, the people around me thought it was terrible, but I felt like I was going through something very important, and I have no regrets about it whatsoever. In fact, I feel like I mastered the anxiety by going through it, getting into it, and then coming out of it."

This phenomenon is very similar to what I observe in patients who are suffering from panic and anxiety. When these individuals allow themselves to feel these emotions in the presence of a therapist and learn tools to master them and be at peace with them, they usually come back from the journey with a sense of mastery. While they may not want to call anxiety and panic "good" feelings, the fact that they now have a sense of mastery and confidence over them is a positive outcome. They are no longer fearful of being blindsided by their emotions again.

Even the most frightening experiences provide the greatest opportunities for learning and can prove profoundly healing when guided properly. By facing your fear head-on, you can conquer it, expand your horizons, gain confidence, and move forward fearlessly.

THE ROLE OF APPROPRIATE PHYSICAL TOUCH

Hunt Priest's story brings up an important caveat regarding the idea of "surrendering" while in a vulnerable, altered state of mind. With a trusted and caring guide, appropriate physical touch can help you process a difficult experience or even accelerate a breakthrough, as in the case of the "laying on of hands" during Priest's trip.

I am a proponent of responsible and appropriate touch when the situation calls for it. I discussed this sensitive subject with Katherine MacLean. She explained:

> So, first of all, we were trained to hold the person's hand. We would practice this with them ahead of time and say, "This is how I'll hold your hand. I will touch your shoulder and ask, 'Would you like me to hold your hand?'"
>
> We prepare people ahead of time so they are ready for that nonverbal contact. That alone is very calming. Safe and consensual nonsexual touch can be very helpful. Again, I'm talking about a shoulder and a hand, nothing else. Holding someone's hand reminds them that it's normal to be feeling what they're feeling. We don't talk about how much time is left or try to distract them. We focus on the fact that what's happening now is safe, and we're with them. We emphasize that it is s normal to be feeling what they're feeling right now, and eventually, this feeling will change. We're going to be here with them as the feelings change.

When I asked MacLean whether she would take patients through a breathing exercise for the anxiety, she says:

I did that with a couple of people. One person was very dissociated, so much so that anything we talked about ahead of time was not going to register. So I held his hand. This was the only time in my experience where I did cross one of those boundaries. I said, "Is it okay if I put my hand on your chest?" because hand holding was not cutting it.

He said, "Yes, I'm okay with that."

I had him breathe into my hand, which was very grounding for him. It got him out of his head and into his body. Once he did that, he kind of woke up and said, "Oh, I'm back, I'm in the room."

In meditation also, where people spiral out into these really high energetic levels and forget that they have a body. Bringing people back into their body is often part of the guide's work. We talked about it with that person afterward to make sure that he was okay. We were all okay, and we addressed the fact that this was an unusual experience.

Handholding and shoulder touching have proven to be effective grounding techniques, not only for individuals undergoing psychedelic experiences but also for those experiencing psychotic episodes unrelated to psychedelic substances. In my practice there have been many times when I have helped people extricate themselves from cyclical obsessive thoughts by simply touching them on the shoulder. Kind human touch is helpful and can be healing.

MacLean says further:

But it also brings up a very important point: how are we going to train people to do this in an ethical way? If touch is one of the things that helps, how do we supervise and hold people accountable to ensure that it doesn't cross a boundary that harms someone? It's a conversation; it's a dialogue. We have to be talking about this now before a large number of doctors and therapists are able to give someone MDMA.

I would like to see advanced consent procedures put in place around the country, which tell the patient in advance, "There might be times when I'm going to hold your hand or touch your shoulder, but I will never, ever touch anything else. I'd like your permission now, in advance, to hold your hand and touch your shoulder." MacLean agrees that giving and receiving advance consent is an excellent procedure. She says:

> Exactly, and we should get consent again during the session. If someone says, "No, I don't want you to hold my hand," we would never intrude.
>
> Even if we know it could help them, we would listen and say, "I'm right here. I'll be here. If you change your mind, I'll be right next to the couch."
>
> Mary Cosimano [a pioneering psychedelic researcher] advises siting on the floor so that we are at the level of the participant on the couch. Instead of being objective professionals sitting back in our chairs, we get down to their level, even lower than them, so that they understand they are in power. They are the empowered person in the room, and we are there in service to them.

SPIRITUAL SURGERY AND ITS RISKS

Sadly, there have been reports of exploitation and misconduct by some treatment facilitators, both in the United States and South America, underscoring the importance of diligently selecting a trustworthy guide. Professional credentials alone are not a guarantee of trustworthiness, although they are a step in the right direction: a credentialing body carefully licenses practitioners.

The actions of a few bad people should not cast a shadow over the transformative potential of these experiences when done responsibly, but you must choose a guide with whom you are prepared to surrender to the experience to gain the full benefit.

As Katherine MacLean explains, "One analogy is the idea of going in for surgery, except the potential risks and benefits with the psychedelic experience are psychological not physical."

When you go into surgery, you cannot insist on remaining vigilant and awake throughout the experience. You must be prepared to surrender to the anesthesia and trust that you are in the capable hands of the surgeon.

She continues, "You want the right kind of medical safety, and the experts who can guide you through those potentially risky scenarios. And then you want to follow up afterward, to make sure that the risks, if there were any lingering effects, have been minimized."

Just as one would not perform surgery on oneself at home, it's ill-advised to navigate the depths of a psychedelic experience without expert guidance.

Psychedelics are extremely powerful substances, and used under proper conditions they are medicines. However, if you take psychedelics at home and guide yourself, best you know in advance that you might encounter powerful emotions including anxiety and panic. Imagine flying a plane for the first time without a teaching instructor sitting at the controls next to you.

"It's a matter of balancing the potential benefits of psychedelics with the acute challenges of working through the experiences and mastering them," MacLean says.

In the next chapters, we will be discussing the work of integrating the insights that are mined during a psychedelic experience.

STEP 7

Integrating the Insights

It was December 1966, and the breathtaking waves were crashing on the shores of Big Sur. I was on the year-end holiday from my faculty position at the University of Michigan. Following an invitation I had flown to Big Sur to study at the newly established Esalen Institute. After three life-changing and enlightening weeks with Perls, I resumed teaching at the University of Michigan. At the trimester's end in April, I drove my Volkswagen Beetle back to Esalen for my four-month summer break.

It was during that period that I met Richard Price, the cofounder of Esalen, and we created my position of Esalen's first resident fellow. This position allowed me to live at Esalen for the next four months in a Round House built over a creek. During this transformative season in 1967, now famously known as the Summer of Love, I studied with pioneering therapists like Dr. Fritz Perls (who founded Gestalt therapy), Virginia Satir (founder of family therapy), and George Bach, (founder of marathon group therapy). Learning about the importance of the therapeutic milieu from British psychiatrist Dr. Ronald David Laing, along with the inspiration from my many experiences at Esalen, was pivotal in shaping my approach to holistic health.

It was at Esalen that I began my study of balneology, the use of natural geothermal waters for healing. These studies culminated in my acquisition of the historic Wilbur Hot Springs and the establishment of what I named The Health Sanctuary. While at Esalen in that summer of 1967 I also had my first experience with ketamine guided by the neuroscientist Dr. John Lily, and massage pioneer Bernie Gunther introduced me to the breathing techniques that would later save my life during my motorcycle accident.

In addition to this immersion in studies on human potential, two other pivotal events occurred that summer. First, I attended the Monterey Jazz Festival where I was exposed to iconic artists like Janis Joplin and Jimi Hendrix. Second, I had my first pure LSD experience, provided by my college roommate Lionel Bloom. Bloom was visiting from his teaching post at the Sorbonne in Paris and brought me LSD from Sandoz, the Swiss pharmaceutical company where Albert Hofmann first synthesized LSD.

At the end of the 1967 Summer of Love, I returned to teaching at the University of Michigan but continued to regularly fly back to Esalen to lead couples' seminars. I also began bringing Virginia Satir's poodle, Colonel, to family therapy sessions. In 1967, I brought Colonel and presented a paper at the Western Psychological Association conference in Chicago, detailing the incorporation of canines into family therapy sessions. This innovative method laid the groundwork for what is now recognized as canine-assisted psychotherapy.

Around the same time, a University of Michigan student introduced me to DMT—N,N-Dimethyltryptamine. Unlike the gradual onset of LSD, one puff of DMT sent me soaring out into the cosmos. I had barely managed to return the DMT-laden cigarette to the ashtray before I was transported to another realm. After ten or fifteen minutes, I turned to my new friend and said, "I want to try that again."

He handed me the cigarette, and I was launched into the cosmos again for another ten to fifteen minutes.

Looking at my friend, I confessed, "I never thought I was the addictive type of person, but I think I'm hooked. I want more of that immediately. Can I have another puff?"

"Sure," he replied.

I took the third puff, and once again I was propelled into an intense cosmic journey. Suddenly, a large, red "CAUTION" sign appeared in the black sky. A voice spoke to me, saying, "Richard, anything that can take you so far so quickly deserves deep respect."

After I came back to this realm, my friend asked, "Would you like another puff?"

"No, thank you," I replied. "I think I've had enough."

I never smoked DMT again.

Later, I realized what was missing for me in that DMT experience. The event happened so quickly that I wasn't able to bring anything useful back, to *integrate* it. I wasn't overwhelmed, which implies a negative feeling. I was just whelmed. It was like I took a rocket ship into space. The visuals were pretty, but it was more like a great rollercoaster ride than the profound inner work I had experienced with LSD during my fellowship at Esalen.

In other words, other than a unique ride, I didn't gain anything useful from the trip.

INTEGRATION, INTEGRATION, INTEGRATION

In 1968, I took a leave of absence from the University of Michigan, moved to San Francisco, and opened the Gestalt Institute for Multiple Psychotherapy on Sacramento Street. In multiple psychotherapy, two therapists were present during all sessions. The two-therapist method was extremely effective but impractical. I have a similar view on having two therapists present for psychedelic therapy. Of course two therapists are far more effective than one but we cannot expect the general public to be able to afford such an extravagance. I believe we need to seek significantly less expensive ways of offering psychedelic treatment, such as group therapy, which we have discussed in this book.

In San Francisco, I lived on Telegraph Hill, close to Coit Tower, and often frequented Enrico's coffee house on Broadway. It was a heady life for me as a twenty-nine-year-old psychologist who, not long before, in school, had been scraping dishes in a sorority house to pay for food.

Instead of returning to the University of Michigan, I took a position at Stanford working with Dr. Irvin D. Yalom on a group therapy experiment. Yalom was studying different group therapy approaches and he chose me, and Dr. Larry Bloomberg, to represent existential therapy. I also began a search for a property with geothermal medicinal water, where I could create a therapeutic community based on what Laing had taught me.

But where could I find a place within a few hours of San Francisco, with natural hot medicine waters, accommodations for overnight visits, and the calming environment of the natural world?

A team of about fifty of us searched the countryside. We were in the right place at the right time. Hot springs had gone out of favor with the advent of prescription medicine. People preferred to pop a pill rather than travel to hot springs. At the time, in the late 1960s and early 1970s, many hot springs were for sale.

Our search team found a hot springs that contained waters like no others. In fact, its slogan was "In all the world, no waters like these."

In 1972, I bought Wilbur Hot Springs and the surrounding 240 acres in Northern California's little-known Colusa County, and created The Health Sanctuary—a safe place to get healthy, which once again became internationally renowned.

Professional realtors talk about the importance of "location, location, location" to distinguish a property.

What distinguishes a professional psychedelic therapist is the after-psychedelic session emphasis on "integration, integration, integration."

While psychedelics can provide profound insights and peak experiences, integration of lessons learned into daily life is required to gain long-term benefits. Psychedelics are not a panacea. The present worldwide enthusiasm for these substances can generate unrealistic beliefs that a single experience will provide a cure-all.

Don Lattin, the author of *The Harvard Psychedelic Club: How Timothy Leary, Ram Dass, Huston Smith, and Andrew Weil Killed the Fifties and Ushered in a New Age for America*, is a proponent of cautious and responsible psychedelic use. He believes that the emphasis on integration differentiates the current psychedelic renaissance from the initial wave of enthusiasm in the 1960s. Lattin defines integration as utilizing the insights gained during a trip to find ways to improve your everyday life and become a more compassionate person.

Lattin quotes philosopher Huston Smith, who noted that the effects of psychedelics are not just about altered *states*, but also about altered *traits*.

Peak experiences alone often do not necessarily bring about change or healing. Instead, the psychedelic journey is shaped by intention, mindset, and environmental setting and integration. Integration is where much of the healing takes place. We gain "altered traits" by reflecting on our experiences, identifying lessons learned, and developing practices to embody them each day.

Furthermore, psychedelic experiences are lengthy and taxing altered states that cannot and should not be induced too frequently. The mind and body require balance for well-being.

Peak experiences, by definition, are temporary; one cannot remain on a peak in an altered state indefinitely. It is inevitable that you will come down from any peak. The question is, how far down will you come and how much will you be able to integrate?

Although the term "integration" has become something of a buzzword, it is essential for gaining lasting benefits from psychedelic experiences and should ideally begin before the psychedelic session itself.

Psychedelics create a period of heightened neuroplasticity, which is the brain's ability to change and adapt, thereby allowing behavioral changes and new perspectives to arise. This is why many psychedelic psychotherapists encourage their patients to set specific intentions beforehand to gain insight into the areas of our life we are most eager to change.

For some, that might be a specific fear around death and dying. For others, it might be a bad habit, an addiction, depression, or an asocial tendency such as social anxiety that we are trying to break free from, as well as other behavioral patterns that no longer serve us.

METAPHYSICAL INTEGRATION

New research is illuminating the mechanisms behind psychedelics' effects on neuroplasticity, yet there is still much to learn about how psychedelics aid in the process of integrating core insights into one's daily life. Psychology and spirituality have attempted to find the language to discuss integration with more precision, but there is another field which might be better equipped to help us understand the underlying framework: philosophy.

During my interview with philosopher Peter Sjöstedt-Hughes, he explained his concept of "metaphysical integration."

Metaphysics is the branch of philosophy that addresses questions about the basic structure of reality. It offers different conceptual models to understand human experiences. Sjöstedt-Hughes proposes the term "metaphysical integration" as using metaphysical perspectives to help integrate psychedelic revelations.

As Sjöstedt-Hughes describes, "People think of philosophy as impractical, ivory tower, theoretical stuff, but there is a practical application of philosophy, or at least metaphysics, to psychedelic therapy."

In his 2023 publication on the topic, Sjöstedt-Hughes notes that leading psychedelic theorists including Dr. Stanislav Grof and Albert Hofmann, clearly saw the need for integration of psychedelic experiences. However, psychology and psychiatry typically do not cover the realm of metaphysics. Sjöstedt-Hughes believes this philosophical perspective can be valuable for psychedelic therapy, especially end-of-life care.

To understand what he means, we must first grasp the distinction between metaphysical and mystical experiences. As we've discussed, mystical experiences involve a sense of unity with a greater reality, often leading to profound personal insights. But the metaphysical perspective goes a step further, attempting to make conceptual sense of such experiences within a philosophical framework.

Ultimately, Sjöstedt-Hughes sees metaphysical integration as advancing psychedelic-assisted psychotherapy to properly meet its subject matter. "If having a metaphysical experience, one should integrate it metaphysically," he explains.

"We are trying to repurpose a tool not designed for the matter at hand—using a hammer to correct grammar. From this perspective, integrating metaphysics is an adjustment that expedites the alignment of the therapy with its subject matter: metaphysics for metaphysical experience."

For individuals facing death, their perception of reality also shapes their sense of meaning and purpose. According to Sjöstedt-Hughes, metaphysical integration can help sustain comfort found through a psychedelic experience by articulating revelations about life and death in a new language—or through an image that goes beyond the limits of language.

As an example, Sjöstedt-Hughes explains: "Let's say you have this oceanic flash, and it causes benefits to your person. After a few months, you might think to yourself, 'Well, that was interesting, but it's obviously a delusion,' and you forget about it and you move on, because you're now reintegrating back into your culture's implicit metaphysics."

However, he notes that if a person is given alternatives through metaphysical discourse, they "might be less likely to let go of that belief and therefore, the benefits could last longer."

As Sjöstedt-Hughes sees it, metaphysical integration provides a conceptual framework to ground insights, so they are not dismissed over time. Though abstract, metaphysics offers comprehensive theories of reality that have been debated for centuries. By understanding these perspectives, we may view profound realizations not as anomalies, but rather as glimpses of established worldviews.

"Even a simple understanding of metaphysics may endow a lasting significance to the person who has undergone an associated metaphysical experience," he says.

To implement this, he has created what he calls the "Metaphysics Matrix," which outlines various positions on the nature of reality. This matrix could give therapists a menu of metaphysical models to help make sense of psychedelic revelations. Patients could resonate with a perspective that fits their experience, adding gravity and meaning to the experience.

While the subjective impact of psychedelics differs, Sjöstedt-Hughes believes this additional philosophical context could enrich the integration process for many. As he notes, psychedelics have been shown to occasion experiences described as metaphysical across cultures.

The metaphysical matrix offers conceptual frameworks, but putting insights into practice requires effort. The real work begins when we return from visionary states to ordinary life.

Though revelations usually come suddenly, their integration unfolds gradually. We must hold truths lightly, yet firmly enough to translate epiphanies into action. Sometimes these realizations come to us through the grandeur of nature or a sudden insight into one of our relationships, only to slip away again later. But we can also capture these moments and make their lessons stick.

This process of intentional insight integration can be illustrated through a personal experience I had during a visit to the home of the Secret Chief, Leo Zeff, in Bolinas, California. Under the influence of 300 micrograms of LSD, I noticed some beautiful flowers that looked particularly vibrant. Struck by their intense colors, I thought to myself, "I want to see the color of these flowers as brightly as this for the rest of my life."

I stared at the flowers for about ten minutes, focusing intently on absorbing their colors into my essence. To my surprise, this simple act of mindful attention had a lasting impact. Since that moment, flowers have consistently appeared more vibrant to me, as if my perception had been permanently altered by that experience.

In a different context, consider the experience of suddenly thinking of someone and feeling a rush of love and compassion for them. How can you sustain this profound feeling?

One helpful method of preserving the experience is to write it down so you can revisit those feelings of love and kindness again later and initiate an open-hearted talk with that person at the right moment. Documenting epiphanies makes fleeting moments eternal.

Each realization, when recorded and later revisited, becomes a strand we weave into the tapestry of our everyday life. Bit by bit, choices sculpt character, and transient moments leave indelible imprints. By integrating insights with intention, we transform revelations into tangible changes in our daily lives.

We must keep and nurture what psychedelics reveal to us, integrating as much of the experience as possible. These metaphysical imprints fill the well from which we draw meaning when death draws near.

HEATHER'S STORY:
INTEGRATION OPPORTUNITY

Heather A. Lee is a breast cancer survivor and certified psychedelic therapist in Colorado whose cancer diagnosis presented a life-changing opportunity in disguise.

"Richard, the week that I got my diagnosis of breast cancer was the week that I became certified as a psychedelic-assisted psychotherapist," Lee tells me. "Well, this is not a coincidence. This is the universe saying to me, here's a place you can be using this medicine with people. Why don't you work on it with yourself?"

Lee's subsequent self-directed experience on a heroic dose of psilocybin took her into a scary place.

"It was dancing with the devil and facing fears and looking at mortality. On that journey, I got this really big download of information that cancer is fear turned cellular. It could even be intergenerational fear from my female lineage, from my mother and grandmother. It was fear-based patterns of thinking around scarcity, money, and partnership, and those absolutely were issues in my mother's life. I could see them as patterns in my life, too. I also got information that I needed to go deep into the wilderness and find sacred water. This is what came to me on my psychedelic journey. I needed to prepare my body for the surgery by going and bathing in this psychic healing water."

Lee trusted the doctors on the medical component of her journey, which ultimately included a double mastectomy and six more related surgeries in a six-month period.

However, she took matters into her own hands when it came to the "psychosocial energetic component" of her cancer—something Western medicine didn't address.

"I was telling my doctors about all of this and they're just looking at me like, 'What are you talking about, lady?'" Lee recalls.

Guided by her intuition, she discovered a camping spot in Lower Elk Falls, Utah, where she found the healing waters she had been searching for since her psilocybin experience.

We got there late in the afternoon and started hiking way into this canyon. The park guide said, "You probably shouldn't go. It's going to get dark. People are heading out now. Not sure about you guys heading in." I said, "No, no, we'll be fine."

When we got to the end of this canyon that we were hiking— gorgeous cliffs on either side, with a stream running through it— there is this waterfall ascending from high, dropping into this clear, crystal blue pool, and there's nobody around.

I was like, "Oh, my God, this is the place. This is the healing water! We have been led here."

I stripped down, jumped in there, and bathed myself in that healing water. I just really felt it was part of my preparation for this surgery and for treating my cancer. I felt like I was doing stuff that was so meaningful to me, so spiritual and energy-based.

Lee's experience speaks to the power of integration, long after an initial "peak experience."

Normally, a person preparing for cancer treatment might find themselves paralyzed by fear—unable to enjoy their travels, let alone find hidden reservoirs of healing in the wilderness. "Although the experience would normally be very fear-inducing," Lee says, "I was still in an incredibly neuroplastic state after my previous journey, which helped me going into the surgery experience."

The cancer removal was followed by a procedure to remove her breasts and have expanders inserted. Unfortunately, one of the expanders became infected and had to be removed, then replaced. After that, she had to undergo reconstruction surgery and a biopsy, for a total of six procedures.

"It was a lot to go through, so I decided not to take any more psilocybin."

During this period, Lee spent her free time doing integration work, which she went on to describe:

Fortunately, I had the luxury to take it easy and spend time resting around the house, intensively working on all of that through cognitive behavioral therapy, guided imagery, meditation, journaling, writing, drawing, and narrative therapy.

I also do something called visual journaling, which I love to do with my clients.

When I sit down to write, I tend to get poetic. [. . .] That's how I express myself. I also tend to doodle and use colors. I make a combination of writing statements, drawing emotions, creating little affirmation statements, and writing poetry. It's a free flow of thoughts that come out in a very visual way.

For me, it's not so much trying to describe what happens on a journey. It's ineffable; you can't really put words to it. When I'm expressing myself on paper, it's not always through words. It's often through images. Even just the act of doodling, or writing a word or a couple of words, puts me back in that state of the emotion that I'm trying to process or the new thought that I'm manifesting and connecting with.

Every day, I did guided meditations with the same music I had used during my journeys. This was a powerful way to do integration, since it allowed me to revisit the same mental and emotional space as before. During these meditations, I would bring myself back into that journey space.

In addition to meditation, I spent a lot of time journaling and working on affirmation statements to reinforce new patterns of thought. I made a conscious effort to notice when I was shifting to fear-based thinking and created new internal dialogue to establish a new default mindset. After a significant psilocybin experience, your brain remains in a neuroplastic state, providing an opportunity to rewire and break free from deeply rooted default modes and thought patterns.

When I attempt to revert to old patterns of fear-based thinking regarding scarcity, money, and partnership, I feel no fear about any of those topics. I am rooted in a place of faith and trust. There is no fear around those things. I have released them.

Like Lee, I've also used drawing, painting, and clay sculpture both during and after psychedelic experiences. Most people who come to therapy, however, are more verbally oriented. A competent therapist can help a patient preserve their insights during the experience just by talking to them. These other nonverbal techniques can be useful if a person is less verbal, and you want another avenue for dealing with their emotions. You can instruct them to paint what they're feeling as a way to capture the essence of some otherwise ineffable experience.

HOW CLINICAL STUDIES HAVE APPROACHED INTEGRATION

Those who think psychedelics promise a quick fix or that a single psychedelic session will resolve complex life issues are liable to be disappointed. Genuine change is difficult work—not a job for shovels but heavy equipment. It takes time and ongoing effort.

However, early evidence is suggesting that for those facing their end of life, a single psilocybin session—followed by multiple integration sessions—can lead to significant alleviation of emotional distress.

In the UCSF study on using psilocybin at the end of life (Woolley 2021), researchers built follow-up integration therapy sessions into the structure of the study to help participants process their experiences, gain insights, and make lasting changes to their lives.

In their study, an initial lower dose of psilocybin was followed by a higher dose, with integration therapy after each to reflect on insights and learnings.

As Andrew Penn, a lead scientist in the study, tells me, "The day after the session we would talk about the experience of the day before. We really try to make sense out of what happened, what was talked about, what was felt."

The trials aim to show how, within the proper framework, a limited number of psychedelic sessions combined with integration can significantly increase quality of life.

The UCSF study was diligent in embedding psilocybin therapy within patients' existing medical treatment. The participants were typically referred by doctors who knew their conditions and histories well. Before the session, their existing medical care team introduced the patient to the psychedelic therapists. Typically, some members of the medical team are involved in the study, and all of them continue the care after the study ends.

This follow-up with the care team creates continuity for patients, allowing insights to take hold and preventing the painful situation that Heather A. Lee found herself in when her surgeons gave her bewildered looks for speaking openly about her psychospiritual healing in the pools of Lower Elk Falls.

AVOIDING THE COME DOWN

The downside of the UCSF model is the expense of psychedelic-assisted therapy conducted by two therapists. Until we create new effective protocols of psychedelic administration, only the super-wealthy will be able to participate and benefit. This is a major drawback of the treatment which must be overcome. Psychedelic group therapy affords one possibility for providing treatment at more reasonable fees.

Heather A. Lee expresses interest in the research and experimentation being done in community, such as group therapy in a retreat setting.

"I prefer to work with this medicine in small groups, creating a container where people can build a little community of support during their experience with these medicines," she tells me.

"Having other people bear witness, hold space for you, share their compassion, and be interconnected can be incredibly powerful. As humans, we have a natural desire for interconnectedness and community. The ancestral roots of these medicines are in ceremony, where people sit in a circle. There is so much power in that practice."

However, Lee fears that in certain circles, group sessions are not followed up with enough integration afterwards.

"I've worked with people who come back from Peru and ayahuasca journeys feeling traumatized, because they have such a big experience and then they hop on a plane and fly back to the States, and there's not that comprehensive integration piece."

I have witnessed a similar phenomenon in my work treating chemical dependence. Many people have gone to famous twenty-eight-day programs and then flown back home with no integration. In fact, in chemical dependency treatment, the therapy which takes place after the residential component is referred to as "after care" as if it takes place after the care. This can unintentionally diminish the perceived importance of the ongoing therapy and support needed after the initial, more intensive residential phase of treatment. Very few people are "cured" after a 28-day program. Ongoing support is typically required for many months or years for a patient to overcome the challenges associated with chemical dependence and the associated lifestyle.

In the 1980s, I established the country's first holistic chemical dependence program called Cokenders Alcohol and Drug Program for individuals struggling with chemical dependence. People from all over the world participated in the program's residential component which I led at The Health Sanctuary at Wilbur Hot Springs. The patients were hardly "new age" and scoffed at new age therapy. Knowing this we offered yoga and called it "stretching," meditation was called "mind clearing," aerobic exercise was called "physical conditioning," nutrition education was called "fuel ingestion," massage was called "bodywork," balneology was called "hot baths," and individual and group therapy was called "therapy."

After completing the five-day residential detox program, patients returned home where therapists awaited them. Upon arrival, a therapist who had trained with me was immediately ready to continue the weekly integration work.

From 1980–1989, I treated 1,500 people in my Cokenders Alcohol and Drug Program, achieving one of the highest success rates in the United States at the time with an astonishing 86 percent clean and sober after a two-year follow-up with patients. We proved to the world that twenty-eight-day programs were unnecessary and possibly driven by deals between hospitals and insurance companies. The Cokenders Program, consisting of five-day residential detox at Wilbur, followed by one and a half years of weekly integration, cost less and was significantly more effective than twenty-eight days in hospital programs. Just as the psychedelic experience, to be fully effective, needs to be followed by integration, the five-day chemical dependence residential needed to be followed by integration. Integration, integration, integration.

Similar to an intense psilocybin or ayahuasca experience, an intensive stay in a rehabilitation facility can be a high experience from which there can often be a later comedown. Patients should be ready and provided with tools to further develop the insights they gained during the peak experience in the subsequent period.

For psychedelics, that's also where integration comes in. How much of the raw material you unearthed can you sift through, polish, and practice? How much of the peak experience are you willing to let disappear into the wind?

During my psychedelic journeys, I've had some fantastic allegorical experiences, from watching the development of civilization at the pyramids in Egypt to feeling connected to every person on the planet and being totally at one with nature. During the time after a psychedelic experience I continue to learn from the insights and need to eat high-octane food, exercise my body, especially my heart, maintain my strength through weight training, breathe clean air, meditate, stretch my muscles, do work with meaning, and spend time with family and friends. Short of these endeavors, I might just sit around with a big silly smile on my face or face the depression of nonmeaning.

Hopefully, the current psychedelic renaissance will not burn out but will transform the culture. For me, it is critical to promote these psychedelic substances as legitimate medicines to drive cultural change. This renaissance comes at a time when millions of Americans have been harmed, physically and emotionally, by ineffective products from Big Pharma. In addition, following the pandemic epidemiologists report that 30–40 percent of the country are suffering from anxiety and depression.

While suffering from a terminal illness may create a greater sense of urgency, there is always a possibility of taking positive steps toward healing and self-enhancement, regardless of how much or how little time each of us has left.

Reckoning with the Afterlife

The notion of eternal punishment understandably breeds deep angst about death. For Hunt Priest, the founder of Ligare whom we met earlier in this book, this fear is not only unjustified from a rational perspective but isn't even warranted by reading the Bible itself.

"It's not scriptural," Priest tells me candidly. "Eternal punishment after death has been used to control people and scare people."

Priest and I both question why so many people profess to believe in a God who created beings only to condemn most to eternal torture.

Yet the threat of hellfire has long been used to instill fear and compel compliance.

When I asked Thomas Roberts about this question, he provided a charitable explanation as to why hell has come to dominate our thinking about death and the afterlife.

"I don't think the church intentionally controls people," he says. "I believe church leaders have deluded themselves into their way of thinking."

However, if you believe in the reality of hell, to what extent is fear of death justified? I argue that there are psychological roots to the fear of hell that are worth examining.

It starts with this: We all make mistakes. In religious language, you can say we're all sinners. Regardless of what you call them—sins, mistakes, missing the mark, or regrets—we all wish we would have done certain things differently. However, once you accept that the past cannot be changed, and you have "sinned," then if hell exists you are going there. Hence the fear of death.

There is one benefit to reflecting on what we're ashamed of or regret, or what we wish we could have done differently.

If we behaved in a way that now makes us uncomfortable, we can benefit from asking: How can I act today so that my behavior aligns with my ethics and values? Examining the past and seeing our errors allows us to choose a different direction in the present. That is valuable.

In this practice, we find something akin to the Christian notion of "repentance"—a poor translation for the actual Greek term *metanoia* used in the New Testament, which refers to a 180 degree change of direction away from those past actions we wish we had done differently. The appropriate response to regret is not fear of hell, but a radical turning toward the values and ideals we wish to embody.

Metanoia is inspired by self-compassion, not self-condemnation. We accept our humanity—that we will always fall short of perfection. But when we realize we've strayed from our values, we recommit to them rather than dwell in regret. This is true repentance: choosing light over darkness, growth over stasis.

Religions often use the fear of hell to deter wrongdoing, but this approach is misguided. Fear breeds little more than anxiety. Dwelling in regret over what cannot be undone serves no purpose. What motivates positive change is connecting with our values and highest aspirations. Letting our highest angels prevail.

ALTERNATIVES TO HEAVEN AND HELL

Peter Sjöstedt-Hughes believes the prevailing black-and-white view about the afterlife fails to reflect the range of possibilities. Sjöstedt-Hughes focuses on philosophers such as Alfred North Whitehead, who argued against binary oppositions or dualisms that limit our view of reality.

"In the West, it seems we have a dichotomy of Christianity or nothingness," Sjöstedt-Hughes tells me. "Annihilationism is also rather scary for a lot of people. That's just nothing."

However, he points out, "Metaphysics comes in and says, 'There are other options here.'"

Sjöstedt-Hughes reminds me that William James, considered the "father of American psychology," also tried to fuse philosophy and metaphysics in proposing a framework for understanding consciousness and mystical experience. According to Sjösted-Hughes, psychology became increasingly empirical and therapeutic, leaving philosophical questions about the mind-body problem unaddressed.

I asked him if he believed life ends at death. He shared his tentative belief in the possibility of eternal life, following philosophers like Baruch Spinoza who viewed time as created by humans. Like Spinoza, Sjöstedt-Hughes takes a pantheistic view that the universe itself is divine.

Sjöstedt-Hughes also shared his experience with 5-MeO-DMT (5-methoxy-N,N-dimethyltryptamine)—a psychedelic compound derived from toad venom, sometimes referred to as the "God molecule"— which gave him a glimpse of what might transcend time.

"I took a high dose of it, by accident," he tells me, adding that it was the closest he ever got to anything that might be related to the afterlife.

"I took it for academic reasons, to discover this timelessness. People always said that the 5-MeO experience is the most unitive one in relation to the mystical text. So, I tried it and analyzed it in terms of that."

Still, he remains agnostic, saying, "You can never be sure. I don't really believe in anything these days. I just entertain different opinions and rule certain things out."

Philosophically, there are two main ways of conceptualizing an afterlife, he explains. Dualism proposes that the soul is distinct from the body, interacting through unknown means. However, dualism fails to overcome the mind-body problem in explaining how something non physical-like consciousness interacts with the physical substrate of the brain. Materialism states that the mind emerges from or is identical to the brain, so when the brain dies, the mind ceases to exist as well—hence annihilationism. But we don't know how consciousness relates to the brain yet.

Sjöstedt-Hughes suggests that the Jewish philosophy of Spinoza, who believed mind and body are one, could provide a framework for believing in an afterlife without dualism or monotheism.

Spinoza's pantheistic view of life deeply resonated with me ever since studying philosophy in college. However, the concept of an afterlife or eternity was beyond my grasp until under the influence of psychedelics I had a powerful vision of death as joining a pink Möbius strip of souls flying through the universe. Would Spinoza call such a vision a glimpse of eternity? This vision opened me to possibilities beyond the big, dreamless sleep of annihilation, though like Sjöstedt-Hughes, I remain agnostic and questioning, ever curious.

REINCARNATION AND EXPANSION OF POSSIBILITIES BEYOND PANTHEISM

While heaven, hell, and annihilation remain possibilities, other views see consciousness as extending beyond the physical body in certain forms. John Buchanan, author of the 2022 book *Processing Reality: Finding Meaning in Death, Psychedelics, and Sobriety*, believes surviving ego death during psychedelic experiences means we "have to die because our brain produces consciousness."

Buchanan recommends the work of the late David Ray Griffin, a pioneer in process philosophy and parapsychology, who describes the possibility of life after death. Griffin examines evidence for phenomena like telepathy, psychokinesis, apparitions, and reincarnation to see if consciousness could exist independently of the body. He concludes that such experiences, along with out-of-body experiences, provide compelling evidence for this view.

Griffin raises the question of whether survival without a body or the ability to act in the world might feel meaningless. However, Buchanan notes that Griffin also suggested that death is the final chapter for some, whereas others who desire to keep being reborn or to unite with the divine can do so.

"We may have choices in death as in life," Buchanan says.

Even if you do not believe in reincarnation in a literal sense, some people find comfort in reframing their death as part of a broader rebirth that occurs in nature at every moment.

Renee Baribeau, author of *Winds of Spirit: Ancient Tools for Navigating Relationships, Health, and the Divine*, spoke eloquently to me about this process of death and rebirth. She says:

If you think about it, these dead leaves that we're talking about are most beautiful when they're dead, especially during a New England fall. The colors come out when they're dead. Moreover, it's the breakdown of that deadness that refuels the next cycle. The leaves break down into their carbon and all of their components, which give life again. I think that's really what religions tried to take from nature: the idea that all that dies is reborn in the spring. You could call it by a different name, but the parts of your body that break down give life to something new. Whether you believe this is your only life or not, you can always give up those parts of yourself to better the earth for the trees that will grow after you. Because we're only here for a short time, there's so much more to learn. If you're really of service, you're always giving yourself to something greater.

CONSCIOUSNESS AFTER DEATH

The belief that consciousness transcends the physical is common in many spiritual and religious traditions. According to philosopher Charles Bush, genuine spiritual and psychedelic experiences lead to the same internal transformation as death. While one is an external act, the other is internal.

Bush believes that while consciousness dwells within and uses the body, it has an inner life of its own where we truly reside. Our rich vocabulary for the mind—imagining, reflecting, and contemplating—describes this inner space where experiences happen, seemingly unrelated to the external world. Although consciousness needs a functioning brain and body, it is not produced by them.

Bush challenges the notion that the brain alone generates consciousness or that altering it necessitates changes in thinking. While brain changes influence thought, so do many experiences. Consciousness itself remains.

"My body and the material world is one aspect of consciousness, but it's not the only aspect of consciousness," Bush tells me. "I have a vast inner life that has nothing to do with my body, my nose hairs, the lake, my computer, or anything else. And it's absolutely real."

Bush sees the nonmaterial and material as equally real, each with its own logic and vocabulary. The inner life and relationships allow us to access a shared consciousness that is otherwise not possible through engaging with external objects alone. In his words: "When you look into my eyes, we are sharing inner consciousness. When I look at the books and bookcases that doesn't happen. Therefore, the nonmaterial exists and is accessible at all times. And it's in relationships where we permeate each other in the same way."

For Bush, death is not the end but a transition to residing full-time in this inner space we already inhabit. "Dying is like losing the usual connection between the physical and nonphysical world we're used to," he says. "Physically, as far as we know, that connection seems lost."

However, consciousness remains—and expands. Out-of-body and near-death experiences show we can access realms beyond the physical even before death.

"Leaving the body is leaving, but it's not that something leaves," Bush explains. "It's just that the region is way larger than the one that you're no longer in anymore. But you were in it before you died."

I remember asking a Catholic priest friend, "You believe that there's something after this form of living?"

He said, "Yes, of course."

I said, "Well, then might you consider changing the name of the ritual called last rites or extreme unction, since you are not really ending, you are transitioning into another form of life?"

While we cannot know what happens after death, some suggest, and others believe, that consciousness transcends the physical in ways intuited through spiritual and psychedelic experiences. We inhabit inner spaces that we call consciousness, and presently, access to these spaces requires a functioning brain and body. However, perhaps death expands our vista, allowing full access to realms that we only glimpse in moments of greatly expanded awareness, some of which are facilitated by psychedelic substances. What remains and what departs during this transition remains one of life's most exciting mysteries.

STEP 9

Living Fully

When I founded the Cokenders Alcohol and Drug Program, described earlier, I began each retreat by telling patients this story:

> Your life of extreme ill health at this point in your addiction has brought you here, to The Health Sanctuary at Wilbur Hot Springs, where you now have the huge opportunity to reorient your life in line with affirming health practices which will enable you to live more fully and even more so than before any addiction or challenging circumstances you've faced. Your addiction may have actually saved your life.

This principle applies not just to chemical dependence but to any serious problem that brings a person to the perspective of needing to get their life act together. Balanced health is not just about reducing drugs and alcohol; it's about how you eat, breathe, exercise, relate to other people, find purpose, and think.

You can apply the same principle to cancer, organ failure, or any of life's problems. Maybe your entire life needs rebalancing, and a diagnosis of a life-threatening disease can create an opportunity to do so.

But before you can begin to start living fully, you must go through a process that begins with acknowledging your condition. If you're suffering from chemical dependence, it means acknowledging it rather than denying it. If you are presented with a terminal illness, that means confronting your mortality as well as living your daily life to the fullest.

Psychedelic experiences can give individuals facing death a newfound appreciation for their remaining life. Journalist Don Lattin noted, from his research into clinical trials, that "many subjects said it really gave them an appreciation for the life they had left to live. It was a real turning point."

While we all have unique intentions in our journeys, there are certain areas that we can all benefit from re-examining from time to time. Psychedelics provide an opportunity to scrutinize both beneficial and descriptive habits to see which actions might better serve us than our current automatic responses.

According to psychedelic scientist and therapist Gisele Fernandes-Osterhold, "The theme of death always brings me in touch with how we're living. This idea that by being aware of our affinity, of our limitations of the time that we're here, the quality of the time in which we're living—it's a constant inquiry into how we're walking and talking in integrity with our heart, in harmony with our relationships, and respecting and honoring the environment, the earth."

It is crucial to understand that stopping a self-injurious habit is only the beginning of starting new healthy habits. This is true for both daily practices and overcoming chemical dependence. For example, the person who is no longer drinking alcohol must also learn how to be a nicer person if they were previously unpleasant while drinking, and they must learn how to nourish themselves with nutritious food that makes them feel positive rather than junk food. Simply stopping an injurious habit is not enough, and this is also true for what we learn from the psychedelic experience. Quitting drinking or using cocaine is only the first step toward a new life.

To support this transformation, I have revised the positive protocol for lifestyle change that I taught my patients in the 1980s. These essential practices promote mind-body health and have enabled me to live fully into my now mid-eighties.

THE 12-POINT PLAN

1. Nutrition

As biochemical organisms, we rely on external fuel for survival. Thus, it is essential to provide the best fuel for our physical functioning and mental well-being. There is a lot of conflicting information available regarding food choices. My recommendation is to keep it simple and select whole, unadulterated foods that are not processed, produced, manufactured, or packaged in cans, bottles, jars, wrappers, or any other kind of container. When you buy packaged food, you are paying for the container, the label, the marketing, and the sales force. Those who manufacture packaged foods know which tastes sell and they manufacture the taste for the sale not for the nutritional value.

This is much less the case with whole foods. Have you ever seen a TV ad for raw asparagus, broccoli, or kale? The rule of thumb is, if the food is advertised or wrapped in anything, think twice before buying it.

To improve your health and mood, focus on eating whole foods, lean proteins, and healthy fats while eliminating or minimizing intake of sugar, salt, processed foods, carbohydrates, packaged foods, and alcohol. Staying well-fueled and hydrated helps to stabilize blood sugar and mood. Choosing to eat meat, poultry, and fish is both a personal decision and a political act. Forests are being decimated to make land for growing grain for cows which provide beef, and fish are contaminated with plastic thrown into the ocean and by industrial fishing.

If you do choose to eat animal products, choosing organic can avoid the intake of various chemicals and plastics, some of which may be carcinogenic.

And, by the way, there is no such thing as "antiaging." Don't buy into the sales pitch of celebrity doctors selling antiaging products. You cannot stop a flower from aging, blooming, and eventually dying. This is true in all of nature. However, what you can do is enhance and even extend your life. The purer the fuel, the smoother the engine runs, be it you or your car.

2. Hydration

Our bodies are made up of about 60 percent water. Drinking an adequate amount of water daily is fundamental to good health, including mood and metabolism. The majority of scientists agree that most people require at least six 8-ounce glasses of water a day, and more when exercising or in warm weather.

Chronic dehydration can affect everything from digestion and circulation to skin health, energy, and mood.

After my heart failure diagnosis, I began to drink my own body weight in ounces of water daily. Did it enhance my health? I believe so, but while I cannot be scientifically certain, I think it was a contributing factor to my rapid recovery and present normal healthy heart.

3. Rest

Proper rest allows for physical recovery, mental rejuvenation, emotional balance, immune system support, and hormonal regulation. Aim for at least seven and a half hours of uninterrupted sleep per night. Do your utmost to sleep in a room without noise of any kind. The shield the body creates to keep out noise uses energy that is better delegated to the immune system.

4. Meaningful Work

The question of whether there is inherent meaning in life is open to debate. However, we all agree that when we ascribe meaning to something, it becomes meaningful. A sense of purpose, whether derived from a career, hobby, or project, provides us with energy. Even constructing a rock wall in your backyard, as Winston Churchill did, can give you meaning and purpose.

To create meaning in your life, I strongly recommend time-blocking or planning your day the night before to provide structure for the day ahead. As I tell my patients, waking up with purpose helps to prevent your day from feeling aimless or empty.

5. Exercise

The body is our transporter through life, and we must never neglect it. We can maintain our body through exercise, rest, food, water, and air. Exercise helps strengthen muscle and bones and build endurance and resilience. Aerobic exercise releases chemicals that improve mood, and studies have shown that these chemicals are among the most effective antidepressants.

I work out on the elliptical machine for fifty to sixty minutes, five to seven days per week. Occasionally, I substitute swimming laps for sixty minutes.

Aerobic exercise is key to conditioning the heart and maintaining an upbeat mood. It involves elevating your heart rate to between 60 percent and 80 percent of its maximum capacity.

To start exercising, I recommend just ten to fifteen minutes of exercise every other day, then gradually increasing the duration by two to four minutes each week. You will soon be able to exercise for sixty consecutive minutes every other day. Once you reach this point, you can decide whether to continue exercising every other day or increase to more days per week.

Although exercise can be challenging if you are depressed or experiencing amotivational syndrome, the benefits to both mood and health make it hugely worthwhile.

Research conducted at Duke University and Consumer Reports has shown that regular aerobic exercise is more effective than prescription medicine for mood elevation and mental health (Babyak 2000).

As we age, it becomes essential to preserve muscle mass because we lose 1 to 2 percent of muscle mass each year after the age of fifty. Maintaining muscle mass is also important for supporting bone density, which can prevent serious injuries from falls. Weight training enhances strength and energy, making it easier to perform everyday activities. A large amount of feeling old is due to loss of muscle mass. Loss of one percent per year adds up to 20 percent loss between age fifty and seventy. Older people feel old because they have literally lost strength.

I started incorporating strength training into my maintenance plan in my fifties as part of my rehabilitation following an accident. Currently, I engage in weight training for three to four hours per week.

6. Stretching

The muscles and tendons are responsible for moving the skeletal system. We feel tension in our muscles, but not in our bones, organs, or blood. Therefore, it's important to keep our "rubber bands" (muscles) flexible and well-oiled to maintain their function.

Keeping the body flexible is also crucial to prevent pain and deterioration. Much of the aging process is the result of tight and dry muscles causing poor posture resulting in pain.

Even light stretching two to three times per week is beneficial.

7. Mind Clearing aka Meditation

Our minds often act as if they want to be the boss or director, but in reality, we are the ones in charge and we direct and use our mind as we wish. As the real boss, we can learn to use our minds as the tools they are intended to be.

Learning to choose and direct our thoughts results in our no longer being at the mercy of our minds. We are not our thoughts, but rather, we are the awareness behind them. Just as our lungs are tools for oxygen intake and our hearts are tools for pumping oxygenated blood, the mind is a tool for cognitive processing.

However, unlike other tools, the brain is so powerful that it can act as if it has a mind of its own. When we allow our brain to take over and be the boss, it can be a wild ride. We never know what thoughts might arise at any given moment. For example, during intimate moments with a partner, we may suddenly find ourselves thinking about work or baseball. Similarly, while focusing on an intellectual or spiritual issue, our thoughts may interrupt us with a compelling message that demands attention or a video of something interesting. These intrusive thoughts and movies can be distracting, uncomfortable, and create anxiety. It is our responsibility to redirect our thoughts to that which we choose to think about.

To control our mind, we can learn to "change the channel" and focus on what we want to focus on, whether it's a subject or simply the present moment. We can choose to focus on our breathing, music, laughter, or anything.

It is imperative that we switch the "off button" and step away from our electronic devices. The must-see documentary *The Social Dilemma* (2020) delves into the dangerous effects of cell phones and social media, featuring insiders warning about technologies they helped build. Unless we carefully control our use of technological devices, we will be glued to them all the time or else at their unavailable mercy.

8. Sexual Activity

Sexual activity, whether alone or with others, is a unique experience that brings about pleasant and exciting sensations like no other endeavor. Orgasm, the climax of sexual activity, and its positive effects on mood can last up to forty-eight hours. Engaging in sexual activity has many benefits such as enhancing health, reducing stress, improving sleep, regulating hormone balance, and strengthening emotional and physical well-being. Sadly, thousands of years of wildly distorted attitudes towards sex, most fostered by the world's religions, has endowed the joy of sexual activity with conflict and guilt. Only through a great deal of hard work, sometimes helped by psychedelic medicine, can we free ourselves from this enculturated straitjacket which constrains us from benefitting from the magnificent gift of sexuality.

9. Community

For the most part, humans are friendly tribal animals who enjoy one another's company. Social connections provide support and shared meaning or purpose. To cultivate these connections, make time for family and friends, join local interest groups, volunteer, or find ways to engage with people outside of your routine social circles. Shared experiences release oxytocin, the "love hormone", which plays a key role in fostering trust and empathy, thereby boosting overall health and happiness. A rich social life can contribute to longevity.

10. Humor

Finding events, situations, and even oneself funny enough to laugh at is a healthy endeavor that brings a feeling of well-being. There are many health benefits associated with laughing, including increased endorphins, decreased stress, increased pain tolerance, improved cardiovascular health, and easier social connections.

Norman Cousins, a distant cousin and editor of the *Saturday Review*, diagnosed with a supposedly irreversible, crippling, and life threatening disease, ankylosing spondylitis, cured himself with humor and wrote a remarkable book, *Anatomy of an Illness: As Perceived by the Patient*. The book—and the healing power of laughter—resulted in

Cousins teaching about laughter as a healing modality at major medical schools. Of the many important teachings in his book is the tactic, allowed by certain conditions, of checking out of the hospital on Friday afternoon and checking back in on Monday morning. Cousin Cousins would check into a hotel for the weekend as he knew the hospital staff was mostly off for the weekend and the food was much better in the hotel. In the hotel he watched funny movies all weekend. It should go without saying that I am not advocating this tactic for conditions where one requires hospital technology or observation.

11. Witnessing

Having the ability to step back and observe our thoughts, feelings, and emotions is a crucial tool for maintaining and expanding self-awareness.

When we witness ourselves, we gain a new and valuable viewpoint that is not accessible when we are completely immersed in our experiences. Witnessing allows us to see options and possibilities in life that we may miss otherwise. Developing the skill of witnessing, of watching and observing ourselves, is a skill that takes a significant amount of time and training and some feel it is worth the effort. A practical and inexpensive method of learning to witness is sitting quietly with eyes closed for five to ten or fifteen minutes each day and watching the inner self. Observe the thoughts and the feelings, closely feeling the sensations in the body, the emotions and the thoughts. What is the nature of the thoughts? Are they friendly, kind, accusatory, happy, sad, angry? These are the thoughts you are producing. Practice witnessing and then choosing your thoughts as they contribute to your emotional state and your life experiences.

12. Gratitude

Expressing gratitude feels good and reminds us that the fact we exist is, in and of itself, an indescribable gift. We have been given the gift of life. We are the product of the fastest sperm and the most receptive eggs. The eggs and sperm that never united continue to exist in nothingness. We are all the chosen ones. As the old fishermen in my gym locker room say, "a bad day above the ground is better than a good day under." Begin each day with identifying something to be grateful for. I endeavor to make gratitude my attitude. On my top ten tool list, gratitude is second only to breathing.

Breathing

Breathing is another essential health tool. Yes, everyone knows how to breathe but not everyone knows the method of breathing that regulates emotions and eliminates anxiety which is called abdominal or controlled diaphragmatic breathing (CDB).

When we experience the fight or flight response, fear, or anxiety, there is a strong tendency for us to tighten our musculature. The same is true when we experience strong emotions. It is as if by tightening the muscles we are creating a protective shield. The unwanted complications of tightening the muscles are that doing so constricts our breathing, raises our blood pressure, and increases our heart rate, all of which contribute to imbalance, discomfort, and impaired cognitive functioning.

Instead of "holding on" and fighting against strong emotional currents we are better served by surrendering to our emotions and fully experiencing them while using CDB to create balance and calmness. The cultural advice to "just breathe," when stressed, is in fact excellent advice.

Breathing is an unusual bodily function in that it is both involuntary and voluntary. Other major functions, such as digestion and blood flow occur without conscious influence. They are managed involuntarily in our vast processing system. Breathing is managed in the unconscious, but we are also able to take control and consciously change how we breathe. Utilizing our dual control breathing system, we can change how we breathe, and we change how breathing affects our bodies. We might apply to breathing the analogy of electric vehicles which can both drive themselves and be driven by us.

So what are the practices required for becoming a skilled CDB practitioner? The answer is the same the man in Manhattan gave when asked how to get to Carnegie Hall, "Practice, practice, practice."

Fortunately, while getting to Carnegie Hall may require years of dedication with fourteen- to sixteen-hour days of practice many times a week, we have an easier task before us with CDB; we can practice anywhere, anytime, and almost anyplace. We can practice CDB standing up, sitting, or lying down, while walking hiking, jogging, or swimming. We can practice alone or with others. But yes, we must practice.

CDB is accomplished by:

1. inhaling from the abdomen for a count of three, making sure that the abdomen expands, and the chest does not;
2. slowly exhaling completely through the mouth for one count longer than the inhalation; and
3. doing whatever it means to you to "let go" and surrender to the moment.

You can practice in brief sessions for a few seconds, for minutes at a time, or even longer. More important than the duration of your practice each time is the number of times you practice. After a certain number of practice sessions, which differs from person to person, you will be able to enjoy the benefits of CDB.

It is an interesting aspect of life that there are times when the simplest solutions are also the most effective. That has been the case in my life when it comes to the treatment modality CDB. So very simple, free of monetary fee, and ultimately effective. CDB can also be *your* lifelong tool, to apply as needed, with no cost other than the time of your life in the practice.

All the health-beneficial activities mentioned above rely on habit formation, which involves practice over time which in turn builds lifelong well-being.

Making small, gradual changes over time through repetition adds up to a great deal. Remember my slogan: a little over a long time is a lot. However, the same principle applies in a negative sense. No one ever decides to drink a quart of alcohol the first time they drink. They start with a small amount and gradually increase the amount over time. This is what I refer to as "the creep". A little something over a long period of time creeps up to a lot of something—whether positive or negative.

Keeping exercise and nutritional intake constant, one soft drink or beer every day adds 46.9 pounds of body weight over a three-year period. Do the math with me: 150 calories × 365 days × 3 years = 164,250 calories, divided by 3,500 calories per pound of body weight = 46.9 pounds gained in 3 years. So the old saying "try it one time; it's not gonna kill ya" is ultimately misguiding.

Start building the fundamental components for balance and health, and within a few years, you will have them all in place. I created this health program in my forties for my Cokenders Alcohol and Drug Program patients, and now at eighty-five, I remain an endurance swimmer and cyclist in excellent health. I am 6 feet 5 inches tall and weigh two hundred pounds with an average heart rate of 65, blood pressure of 113/68, blood oxygen level of 98, a typical body temperature of 97.8, and LDL cholesterol less than 150.

THE SYSTEM WORKS

Prior to performing the wide excision and lymph node sentinel biopsy to determine whether my malignant melanoma had metastasized, my distinguished UCSF surgeon, Dr. Jonathan George, informed me that I should not expect results for about a week. However, two days later, on a Saturday morning, he called me with the results.

"Richard, you're clear," he told me, "There's nothing in the lymph node."

How had this cancer that often kills in six weeks spared me for what was then already a year since first noticed? Dr. George credited my immune system for building a protective capsule and stopping the spread of the cancer.

The concerted efforts to live well—eating clean, reducing stress, engaging in meaningful work, and using the described health tools—had strengthened my immune system to overcome adversity.

With the cancer threat removed, I focused fully on my heart. The cardiologists advised halving my exercise but instead I decided to double it, increasing my cardio exercises to six to seven days a week. I drank half my weight in ounces of water each day and cut my already low alcohol intake by 97 percent, enjoying only the occasional Rasputin beer to celebrate certain occasions. My organic plant-slanted diet grew stricter. I regularly microdosed LSD, aiming for once weekly, to facilitate neuroplasticity and gaining new insights.

Six months after the heart failure diagnosis, tests showed my left ventricle pumping an ejection fraction of 55 percent—normal. Another six months later it was still 55 percent. At eighteen months, it was 63 percent—better than before this brush with failure had begun.

I do not claim that psychedelics healed me. In fact, I was careful to limit my usage due to the known potential heart risks associated with MDMA, LSD, and psilocybin.

Rather, I credit my ongoing work of integrating a lifetime of health practices with psychedelic experiences to create an anxiety-free recovery.

Dying Gracefully

Aldous Huxley, the renowned English writer, philosopher, and psychedelic explorer, spent the final months of his life in a state of unremitting pain and distress. In a letter to his brother Julian, Aldous's wife, Laura, described her husband's deteriorating condition and unceasing suffering in the days leading up to his death:

> There is so much I want to tell you about the last week of Aldous' life and particularly the last day. What happened is important not only for us close and loving but it is almost a conclusion, better, a continuation of his own work, and therefore it has importance for people in general.

When Laura wrote of the continuation of his work, she was alluding to her husband's mission to aid humanity in "opening the doors of perception"—in large part through the conscious use of mind-altering substances.

Ten years after publishing his psychedelic autobiography *The Doors of Perception*, Huxley found himself on his deathbed. He had been battling laryngeal cancer for nearly a year, and despite rounds of treatments and a regimen of heavy medications, his condition continued to worsen. The disease had spread too far.

Huxley, who was unable to speak, scrawled a note on a tablet to Laura, who was attending his bedside: "Try LSD 100 intramuscular."

Huxley was asking Laura to administer him a sizable dose of his favorite psychedelic medicine to relieve his distress in a way the narcotics could not. He was hoping to gain "moksha"—a transcendent, mystical insight into the nature of existence—one last time before passing.

Though radical, Huxley's request was not unfounded. He had spent decades researching psychedelic compounds and believed firmly in their potential for providing transcendence—even up to and including the passage into death itself. In his final moments, Huxley wanted to test this hypothesis for himself. His vision went far beyond his era's thinking, yet he saw what we are now only beginning to grasp—that these powerful molecules may relieve anguish for the dying in a way conventional medicines can't.

MAKING PEACE AT THE NEW BEGINNING

Our journey towards acceptance of death began with the topic of avoidance. Along the way, we have sought to reframe dying as an opportunity to make the most of our remaining time. But as the hour of death draws near, the nature of that acceptance begins to shift. Once we reach the point of being incapacitated or *non compos mentis*—not of sound mind—we shift our attention to the topic of dying with grace, peace, and dignity.

Renee Baribeau says, "A lot of times, when people are really suffering about their death, they're not open to exploring the fact that they could have a death with their last exhale out being the one of freedom."

We cling so tenaciously to life that we fail to realize death's release.

John Ivey, a terminal cancer patient who was brave enough to speak openly about his sub-rosa psychedelic experience, sees death as a "passage through God." Ivey describes his view of death to me, following several powerful psychedelic experiences, stating, "We're talking about using plant medicines as well as other forms of meditation to move the consciousness into a realm that recognizes that the three times, the past, the present and the future, all exists now."

He continues, "I am engaging in a process of looking down the road to meet the opening. For me, this happens when I get rid of this decaying meat body."

Ivey saw death as a liberation and worked to prepare his consciousness for this transition.

Although he didn't know when his last breath would arrive, Ivey was determined to "die consciously."

"At some point," Ivey says, "I will have to lay down and say, 'No, I will not take Oxycontin. I don't care how much pain is coming. I'm not going to die unconsciously.'"

He notes that he is approaching his death as a "sadhana"—a spiritual practice in Buddhism.

"I am approaching that moment when I will be liberated from this physical body. The movement at that point, when the physical body stops and the consciousness moves forward, is the moment that I am working to prepare for."

But we need not prepare alone. In addition to family and friends, there are healthcare professionals who can aid in this work—what Catherine Durkin Robinson referred to as the "very real work" of dying.

The primary task of this final preparation might be overcoming our fear of the actual dying itself.

Hospice nurses frequently encounter patients gripped by this fear. Julie McFadden, a hospice nurse and popular medical educator, told me that around 70 to 80 percent of her patients express fear about death when entering hospice care.

However, she clarified, this does not mean that they are living fully in fear.

McFadden found her life's calling in hospice nursing. After years of working as an intensive care unit (ICU) nurse, struggling to keep patients alive, she grew weary of prolonging suffering.

"Man," she tells me in an interview, speaking of her time as an ICU nurse, "we need to do this in a different way. I can't keep doing this day in and day out. It was really taxing on me, and I just wanted to be a part of something different."

During the time she was still working as ICU nurse, she jumped at the chance to work in hospice care—applying for a job that listed previous hospice experience as a requirement.

"I didn't have that, but I just thought, 'I'm going to try it,'" she recalls.

"I got the job and here I am, many years later, working in hospice."

A born educator, McFadden began sharing insights from hospice work to combat misunderstandings around death and dying.

Her friends urged her to spread the message, saying, "You need to tell people about this. People don't know this stuff and you're good at explaining it. You should start a podcast or something."

During a family visit, McFadden found her nieces engaged with the social media platform TikTok. Though unfamiliar with the app, McFadden saw an opportunity.

"I'm going to try that," she thought. "I'm going to make videos about death and dying and see what happens."

One of her videos went viral, and as of this writing, she has over 1.4 million followers on TikTok.

Through educating others, McFadden fulfills her calling to ease people's suffering at life's end. On social media platforms such as TikTok and Instagram, she builds connection and community surrounding experiences many shun discussing.

"I love connecting with people," she tells me. "I love the time I get to spend with people."

For McFadden, hospice work becomes a labor of love, focused on life's most meaningful moments.

McFadden finds that openly discussing death helps alleviate distress.

"Talking about it—and even just saying things like, 'I'm afraid to die,' 'I don't want to die,' or, 'I'm sad to die'—leads to acceptance."

We must give voice to fears about death to be able to overcome them.

An Example of Making Peace

Gisele Fernandes-Osterhold's training as a psychotherapist enabled her to have conversations with her grandmother about death when she was approaching the end. As Fernandes-Osterhold tells me:

My maternal grandmother was eighty-six years old, and I went to visit her in Brazil. It was the very last time I saw her and I knew that she had a tumor in her lung and she would die sometime soon. . . . She told me she was afraid of dying. And I asked her what exactly she was afraid of? And she said, "I'm afraid of having trouble breathing." She knew it had to do with her lungs.

She said, "I'm afraid I won't be able to breathe."

I listened to her, and we talked about it. I validated her fears. I said, "Are you afraid?"

She said, "No."

"Are you afraid of leaving the people behind?"

She said, "No."

Her fear was just the transition.

Fernandes-Osterhold comforted her grandmother:

"Okay, so if that's what scares you most, how exactly would you like to die?"

Her grandmother replied, "I would like to die like a birdie. I would just go to sleep and die peacefully."

Fernandes-Osterhold promised to hold her grandmother in her "heart and prayers" for this wish to come true, easing her distress. She gave her grandmother an opportunity to voice this fear, validating it and comforting her. By discussing death openly and planning the death she wished for, Fernandes-Osterhold's grandmother gained peace in her final days.

THE PLACE FOR HOSPICE & PALLIATIVE CARE

In the mock patient interview with Catherine Durkin Robinson, my "doula for a day," I discovered my reluctance to consider hospice care for my "last lap." When she asked my thoughts on hospice, I replied, "Something to keep away from as long as possible, because you go to hospice when you have a prognosis of six months or less."

I used to see hospice as a place one goes to when all hope is lost, though Durkin Robinson clarified:

"Well, you certainly could, though most hospice organizations will take patients who have twelve months or less [to live]."

Though hesitant to consider hospice, I knew precisely how I wished to die: at home, surrounded by loved ones. To achieve this, I would take matters into my own hands.

I told Durkin Robinson, "I decided in my twenties to take control of my dying when I lost my best friend, Alan Pinsince, who was suffering from glomerulonephritis, and he took himself out. He got to the point where life was not worth living and he overdosed on pills."

Alan's death has shaped my views; I acquired morphine sulfate pills just in case I ever "needed" them, and I have had the pills with me ever since. If I ever find myself in a condition where I know it is time to go, I will plan and implement my departure instead of burdening others.

Siobhan Greene, who leads the Hospice Giving Foundation, clarified the difference between palliative care and hospice. In short, palliative care provides coordinated support through illness while hospice delivers comfort at life's end, foregoing aggressive potentially life-saving treatments in favor of easing the dying process.

Greene explains, "Together, the family, the patient, and the doctors and nurses have come to the understanding that this illness will very likely result in the death of this person, and more medicines, treatments, and interventions are not necessarily appropriate any longer."

In other words, hospice delivers compassionate care, managing pain and meeting psycho-social needs.

"Palliative care is an approach to medical care with a team of professionals when somebody has a very serious illness," she says. "The term we use very strongly in that discussion is 'serious illness.' Somebody does not have to have a terminal diagnosis to receive palliative care."

Greene advises coming to palliative care when "you get a diagnosis of a very serious illness. Say you have a diagnosis of Parkinson's [disease].

People can live for twenty or thirty years with Parkinson's, but it's a very serious illness and it's going to take its toll on your body."

For illnesses like Parkinson's disease or ALS (Amyotrophic Lateral Sclerosis, a neurodegenerative disease), palliative care helps navigate difficult choices and secure necessary support.

"The palliative care team is brought in to help pull together all the different aspects of the person's illness and develop—with that person and their family—a goal of care," Greene says.

They determine best options for treatment, easing transitions between home and hospital.

Some utilize palliative sedation, which involves the use of medication to reduce consciousness and alleviate severe, refractory symptoms that cannot be adequately controlled by other means. This can include pain medication but may also involve sedatives or other drugs to manage symptoms such as agitation, delirium, or respiratory distress. In certain cases, patients may choose medical aid in dying to experience a "compassionate passing."

Julie McFadden clarifies for me that in states with "Death with Dignity" laws like California, people can end their own life if they meet certain criteria. These criteria typically include being terminally ill with a prognosis of six months or less to live, being mentally competent to make decisions, and being able to self-administer the prescribed life-ending medication. The patient must also make multiple requests for the medication, both verbally and in writing, with a waiting period between requests.

For those not wishing to pursue such extraordinary measures at life's end, medical aid in dying provides a means of navigating the dying process on one's own terms.

Dr. Ira Byock, former director of Palliative Medicine at Dartmouth-Hitchcock Medical Center and author of numerous books on palliative care, spent three years writing his seminal book *The Best Care Possible: A Physician's Quest to Transform Care Through the End of Life*. In it, Byock argues for a personalized, compassionate approach to end-of-life care, tailored to meeting individual patients' needs rather than taking a one-size-fits-all approach.

"The best care," Byock says, "involves making the best medical diagnoses and [using the best] therapeutics and then applying them in a highly personal fashion to one's personal priorities and values. It brings an interdisciplinary team approach to people's physical, emotional, social, interpersonal, and spiritual well-being during the course of an illness."

To illustrate his approach to personalized care, Byock shared a story from the book about Sharon, a teenage girl with severe cystic fibrosis, whom he treated at Dartmouth-Hitchcock. Sharon was reluctant to engage with hospital staff during frequent stays, but Byock made it his mission to connect with her. He discussed her dream of becoming a veterinarian and helped arrange for her to meet her celebrity crush, the "Animal Planet" TV host Jeff Corwin. This transformed Byock and Sharon's relationship and she later told him the day she got to meet Corwin was the best day of her life. By focusing on Sharon's quality of life and seeing her as an individual, Byock provided compassionate care beyond mere medical procedures.

Although none of Byock's books mention psychedelics, he did tackle the subject in a 2018 article published in the *Journal of Palliative Medicine*, entitled "Taking Psychedelics Seriously."

"After nearly fifty years of watching research on the topic evolve," he tells me in an interview, "I thought it was time to come out and say it's time for us to take psychedelics seriously."

However, he remains guarded against sensationalist claims about their efficacy, noting we must proceed carefully. In our conversation, Byock speaks of the dynamic change in healthcare, with positive and negative events happening concurrently. On one hand, he says the science of palliative care continues advancing beautifully, with research into areas like symptom management and measuring patients' quality of life. On the other hand, Byock argues, palliative care is not immune to the "pervasive greed" defining American medicine today, citing the rise of for-profit hospice and palliative care models. Those looking to integrate psychedelics with for-profit medical clinics would be wise to heed his warning about the greed built into the system.

HONOR THY DAUGHTER:
THE MARA HOWELL STORY

Discussions of palliative care and hospice can often seem abstract, especially for those who have not personally experienced a serious illness or are at the end of their life. Many of us fear dying in hospitals, as we may view these places as prioritizing aggressive treatment over a peaceful end of life. The healthcare system can be a difficult environment when life is on the line, and it may not always seem like a compassionate place for those who are approaching the end of their lives.

In 2011, I interviewed Marilyn Howell about her daughter Mara's death from cancer at just thirty-five years of age. When the medical system failed her, Mara finally found relief in MDMA-assisted psychotherapy, though no legal options existed at the time. Her story reveals the quest for purpose that drives us, and love that lifts us up when our days hold more pain than joy.

I am reproducing my full conversation with Marilyn here because the story has touched my heart and that of thousands of my listeners as it relates to the power of psychedelics to alleviate end-of-life distress.

Dr. Richard L. Miller: For those of you just tuning in, we're talking to Marilyn Howell about her book *Honor Thy Daughter.*

Marilyn, tell us about when you first learned of your daughter Mara's illness.

Marilyn Howell: Certainly. My daughter had been experiencing abdominal pains for months and had gone to her own physician in Oakland, California. They were suspecting endometriosis. She didn't tell me how bad the pain was. She didn't want me to worry.

They used a less expensive option than a colonoscopy—a sigmoidoscopy—that didn't reach far enough when they actually had a scan showing there was a problem.

She didn't tell me this.

Since she was an adventure world traveler, I thought perhaps she picked up some kind of tropical disease—parasites, whatever.

On her way back from a diving expedition in Honduras, she stayed with me in Boston, and really let me know that she was hurting. When she started bleeding, I insisted that she go to the emergency room. That's when she finally had the colonoscopy.

Dr. Richard L. Miller: How much later from the original testing was this testing when she got the call?

Marilyn Howell: Seven months later.

Dr. Richard L. Miller: It's seven months after the original testing and they perform a colonoscopy and you find out that . . .

Marilyn Howell: It's a huge mass, and she needs surgery right away. When she had that surgery, not only was that mass cancerous, it had spread beyond the colon. The physician had to remove her spleen, part of her pancreas, twelve lymph nodes and most frighteningly of all, was the very suspicious looking lymph nodes behind her aorta that he couldn't reach.

Dr. Richard L. Miller: I'm now going to shift from talking to Marilyn Howell and ask Marilyn, speaking as a mom, a question. Mom, you were there when she received this diagnosis. What was it like for you emotionally, as a mom?

Marilyn Howell: I went into a kind of shock after hanging up the phone when the surgeon told me all that he had done. My body started spasming, and I collapsed on the floor, jerking and thinking that I was going to die. I suppose that's when people have that broken heart syndrome when they die, but I didn't die.

I managed to call Mara's dad, and we went to the hospital. He went into executive functioning, and since I knew a great deal about medicine, that became my area to help. The way that her father worked out his anger and frustration was to try to pursue a lawsuit, which went nowhere because ultimately, they couldn't prove that there would have been a different outcome had they done the right test.

Dr. Richard L. Miller: What happens next? Mara is in Boston with you. She has had these operations. You've talked to the doctor, and then what?

Marilyn Howell: The only real options that mainstream medicine have are surgery, chemotherapy, and radiation.

What was recommended for her was, at that time, the gold standard for colon cancer, a chemical cocktail and radiation. But even then, she was told that only one third of patients respond.

Her first response is to cry, "Oh my God. This is like a death sentence. Why don't I just let cancer do its thing?"

That was her first reaction. Within a few days, she became a very strong willful young woman.

She said, "I'll do the chemo. I'll do whatever it takes to beat this thing."

That was the stance she took until three weeks before she died, in spite of how weak and sick she became, in spite of how many protocols [were implemented]—four at the minimum, two she couldn't complete because she was sick. She would have done anything to survive.

Sometimes, her decisions were not the same ones I would have made, but I was determined to support her wishes no matter what.

Ultimately, all the chemotherapy turned out to be agonizing and shortened her life.

The chemotherapy was highly ineffective, and each one debilitated her more. That's the nature of chemotherapy. Are you going to kill the cancer before you kill the patient?

I couldn't find anybody who knew anyone with the late-stage cancer that she had that survived more than five years. She was really fighting a losing battle, but the determined person that she was, besides the mainstream options that she wasn't willing to bypass, she had acupuncture, various herbs, and at one point she received little brown pills from a doctor Dhonden, who had once been the private physician of the Dalai Lama.

One of our huge adventures together was to go to Abadiânia in Brazil, the town where John of God is said to do his miracles. She actually went back there again on her own—to this incredible healing community. We had heard so many miracle stories. She saw some amazing things when she was there, but we didn't know that there were limitations on what could be done. She was too sick for what he called "invisible surgery."

Dr. Richard L. Miller: This is the man who also does what's called invisible surgery, João de Deus in Abadiânia, Brazil.

Marilyn Howell: Yes. Which is, I suppose, faith healing. Our attitude going into it was, let's give this our full attention. I suppose my own feeling was that it was like an amazing community of placebo effects with love and healing and support, meditations, all these good things going on. I don't know to this day whether John of God himself has any particular healing powers.

Dr. Richard L. Miller: I know that the placebo effect is powerful and can potentially have a positive effect. Questions worth asking are: how much benefit, for how long, and at what cost?

Can you tell us about the center in Chicago that you came across?

Marilyn Howell: That was a very unfortunate experience. John of God didn't cure her, but the experience was uplifting and positive.

Dr. Richard L. Miller: John of God also didn't charge her $75,000 for a month.

Marilyn Howell: Some of that was the hospital fees. It was a combination of a whole lot of things. It felt very exploitative. She had already been through four chemotherapy protocols.

The original idea, since it was an integrative center, was to get her body strong and able to handle more treatment.

They didn't get her body strong. She was in a pain crisis.

While we were there, she had a celiac nerve block procedure, where they injected alcohol into the spinal nerve to kill it, hoping that that will also kill the pain. That didn't work. It was horrific. They also tried an intrathecal trial. That's lacing a tube that goes in towards the cerebral spinal fluid so that they can deliver medications more efficiently. That failed.

Dr. Richard L. Miller: Oh my gosh, and what is it like for you both psychologically as you are going through these brutal experiments on her body?

Marilyn Howell: Absolutely hell. I would say that the only thing that kept me from wishing I would die is that I couldn't abandon Mara.

Because the pain medications weren't working, they thought, "Well, let's take off all these fentanyl patches. Let's see if morphine will work."

Morphine had no effect whatsoever on her pain. She was writhing in agony. All they could say is keep upping the morphine until it got to a place where it would have killed her if she took more. She had to writhe it out until they could try something else. Pain management took over our lives.

Dr. Richard L. Miller: I can feel my blood boiling hearing this story. I want to know who they are, and how I can expose them and save other people from them, but I won't do that. Instead, I come back here to be present with you. I can feel what David, your husband, must have been feeling as these people are performing these failing medical procedures on your daughter and charging very significant sums of money at the same time. It sounds so agonizing. At the same time, you had to focus on the young lady and her life.

Where did you go next?

Marilyn Howell: Well, fortunately, we have wonderful friends who transformed my teaching studio into a hospital room. They arranged for hospice care. None of which Mara was willing to do except for the fact that she needed twenty-four-hour pain management.

She said, "Okay, I'll come home, but I'm not coming home to die. I'm coming home for pain management, get that under control. Then I'm going to enter clinical trials in Boston."

She was serious through all of this in all her agony and all her pain. I can't even think of all the medication she took—from Norco to fentanyl to the failed morphine, back to fentanyl, then to methadone. The doses of methadone kept going up and up and up. She had anti-anxiety [medication] and antidepressants, anti-psychotics, anticoagulants, and anti-inflammatory [medicines].

Fifteen medications at one time; they kept shifting but nothing was working. At the point where she was getting heart palpitations because the methadone doses were getting very dangerously high, the attending nurse was at her wit's end.

There happened to be a friend who sent me, sometime earlier, a note about a research project that was being proposed at McLean [Hospital], Harvard, very near to us, for anxiety and depression in advanced-stage cancer patients. The protocol might have some effect on pain. My difficulty in presenting that to Mara was that it was for end-stage cancer patients, meaning terminal.

Dr. Richard L. Miller: Was that the MDMA study?

Marilyn Howell: This was the MDMA study and, indeed, they called it advanced cancer now. They don't use terms like terminal or end-stage anymore. They've learned.

Dr. Richard L. Miller: MDMA, or methylenedioxymethamphetamine, is a medicinal empathogen, also known as a recreational drug called ecstasy. It is extremely important to differentiate between the medicinal use of a chemical or a plant and its recreational use. In this case, we are discussing medicinal use. Please take us through this, Marilyn.

Marilyn Howell: Thinking that maybe there was hope, maybe I could get Mara into that Harvard study, maybe something would address her pain, not to mention her anxiety and depression, I called Dr. John Halpern, who is the lead investigator. He told me the FDA had approved the study, but the DEA was still having them go through more hoops. He didn't think it would be ready in time for my daughter.

He did tell me about MAPS, the Multidisciplinary Association for Psychedelic Studies, and that perhaps they were aware of some other alternative clinical trials. That proved not to be a fruitful place to go as there was nothing else available at the time.

I'm very determined at this point. My daughter is suffering. She's at risk from dying from the pain medications before she dies from the cancer.

I decided that underground therapy was the only option I have left. How could I find an underground therapist? How could I find the MDMA?

I was also aware that there had been successful treatments with psilocybin for very ill, end-stage patients. I sent the word out via email to everybody I knew and everybody Mara knew. It only took us a week, through the grapevine of people, and we found someone who was the ideal person to do the co-therapy with me. There's usually a male-female team when psychedelic therapy is done.

We found this amazing person who had sat many sessions with people, who believed that MDMA could help Mara.

About three months before her death, she had her first session with MDMA, and her first experience in many, many weeks, without pain, with a sense of interest and curiosity and pleasure, even the beginnings of being able to talk about her cancer in a little bit more open way.

Dr. Richard L. Miller: You are a Harvard-trained scientist telling us that your daughter was given just about every drug known to modern medicine, and none of them relieved her pain, which came from cancer, until you managed to get her MDMA, which did relieve her pain for the first time. Did I get that right?

Marilyn Howell: You got it exactly right. I might point out that what persuaded Mara, since she didn't want to have anything to do with end-of-life treatment, was the fact that psychedelics can produce mystical experiences—transformative experiences—sometimes even miraculous healings. It was really for the potential of tapping into some kind of transcendent state and healing that she did it. That was Mara's goal.

A miracle would have been wonderful, but since I had pretty much given up, I just wanted her out of pain. I wanted some kind of acceptance to take place. I didn't want her death to be a horrific fight.

The MDMA therapy was a way of meeting our very different but compatible goals in this case. Mara's need for some potential healing and relief of pain, my hope that through the therapy, she could gain some acceptance and not fight and suffer so much.

Dr. Richard L. Miller: How many more MDMA experiences did she have before she was administered LSD?

Marilyn Howell: She had one more experience with MDMA, which again, was a very positive experience. It wasn't anything miraculous. She wanted something that was going to change the game. We decided to try psilocybin. It's amazing how little effect it seemed to have. When marijuana was added, that seemed to bring on the effect. She was able to start talking about her disease, what her feelings and thoughts were. It opened a window to her unconscious mind.

Dr. Richard L. Miller: With the MDMA she was able to open up. What effect on the pain level did the combination of marijuana and psilocybin produce?

Marilyn Howell: The pain level was better, but the way she described it with the marijuana was that the pain is still there, but it's not me. She felt a distance from it. It wasn't the whole of who she was. She could be a person and have this pain. That was really the beginning of using marijuana more regularly.

She would joke that I was her "mom bong." If I took cool sips of water, I could take in the smoke and then blow it into her, like a vapor.

Dr. Richard L. Miller: Did the marijuana alone give her relief from pain?

Marilyn Howell: It helped. The side effects were considerably less than the other pain medications that she was on.

Dr. Richard L. Miller: Marilyn, we're running out of time. Please take us to the LSD experience.

Marilyn Howell: The LSD. Remarkably, she had 300 micrograms, which is quite a whopping dose, but it did not do very much at all, so we added MDMA and marijuana.

Again, she had another period of time where there was relief, where it felt like she had a bit of life back, but she was very, very ill at that point. There was no transcendent experience at that point, which was just a few weeks from death.

She knew that she wanted to go back to MDMA one more time, to be out of pain and to love life. There still could be some positive experiences left for her. Indeed, her last two experiences, which were with MDMA, two days before she died.

Dr. Richard L. Miller: And they were positive experiences?

Marilyn Howell: They were amazing experiences.

Dr. Richard L. Miller: Did she go out and transition under the influence of MDMA?

Marilyn Howell: She did indeed. On the very last day of her life, she only woke up enough to say yes, she wanted MDMA. What it did from the perspective of her father and I looking at her is, it took away the convulsions and tics, the labored breathing.

She was just sleeping peacefully. At the very end, after she'd been apparently sleeping for hours, I picked up Laura Huxley's *This Timeless Moment*—something that was just like an impulse. I needed to do something, find some source of wisdom, and I began to read to her about passing. When a person is in that state, we often don't know if they can hear us, if they're conscious, but sometimes they're very much aware. Laura Huxley spoke about the importance of touch and the human voice in helping someone pass this time of loneliness onto the other side.

Dr. Richard L. Miller: You read Laura Huxley's account of her husband, Aldous Huxley, transitioning to death under the influence of LSD.

Marilyn Howell: Yes, but we didn't get that far. I just got to the part about voice and touch and acceptance. As I read that part, Mara, who had been asleep (and I thought perhaps she would never wake up) took her hand out from under the covers, reached across, put her hand in her father's palm, turned her head to look at him, had this expression of tremendous peace and joy, and took her last breath.

It was her last gift to us, to let us know that she was aware we were there. We were accepting her. We were helping her on her passage, and that her passing was one of peace and love.

Dr. Richard L. Miller: Marilyn, I thank you from my heart for sharing your touching story.

Marilyn Howell: Thank you, Richard.

Howell's poignant story highlights an important point—those facing terminal diagnoses are extremely vulnerable. In desperate times, it is understandable to grasp at any strand of hope. However, we must remain vigilant against manipulative charlatans who would exploit that vulnerability.

John of God—now eighty-one years old—whom Howell visited, was one such predator. He will live out the rest of his days in prison, after facing over six hundred accusations of sexual abuse.

Desperation can cloud judgment, but we must not let it render us blind to evil. There are ethical avenues of spiritual healing and hope. The ailing deserve so much better than to have their last days darkened by deceit and abuse when they are at their most defenseless.

May this serve as a somber reminder: we must care for the vulnerable and be vigilant stewards. Our shared humanity calls us to expose the merciless who would exploit, not uplift, those navigating life's most difficult passage.

Aldous Huxley's final days mirrored Mara's suffering, as pain and medications gradually robbed him of his former vitality and mental clarity.

Like Mara, Huxley was a fighter to the end. He knew death was near but clung to hope of recovery.

Laura Huxley noted, "He thought he might be so sick for another three or four weeks, and then he could come back and start his normal life again. This fact of starting his normal life occurred quite often."

Also, like Mara, Huxley sought transcendence through psychedelics when all else failed.

Huxley's final moments were marked by an easing of anguish through Laura's loving support. After administering the first 100 micrograms of LSD to her husband, Laura felt a sense of relief in seeing his own relief.

She knew "what was to be done." She gave Huxley another dose, sitting by his side. "Darling," she asked, "would you like me to take it also?"

Though unsure herself, Laura remained present for Huxley.

Laura noted changes in Huxley's face as the LSD took effect, though when asked if he felt it, Huxley said no.

"Yet, I think that something has taken place already," Laura wrote.

Huxley had "accepted the fact of death; he had taken this moksha medicine in which he believed."

He enacted his vision from his final novel *Island,* where residents of Pala learned to accept death peacefully under the influence of moksha-medicine.

As Huxley's breathing slowed, Laura spoke words of comfort: "go, go, let go, darling; forward and up. You are going forward and up; you are going towards the light."

She repeated this message for hours, taking breaks when overcome.

She saw "the beginning of struggle in his lower lip," but her words seemed to ease him.

"There was absolutely not the slightest indication of contraction of struggle," she writes.

Huxley's breathing began to slow, until bit by bit, it ceased.

Laura recounts this exit as a gradual process—not a sudden departure of the spirit with the final breath. There were no convulsions, no drama. The testimony of several witnesses confirmed the serene beauty of his passing, and yet Laura still wondered if she had imputed this serenity to his experience out of wishful thinking and desire to fulfill his literary prophecy.

"If the way Aldous died were known, it might awaken people to the awareness that not only this, but many other facts described in *Island* are possible here and now," Laura wrote.

Huxley's death reveals we need not suffer life's end alone and afraid. By accepting death while seeking transcendence, Huxley died with his dignity intact. Releasing the ego, we can all open to this timeless awareness.

The stories of Mara Howell and Aldous Huxley reveal the possibility for dignity and peace at life's close. By letting go of fear and embracing compassion, we can ease death's passage for ourselves and others. Our lives thus find meaning in awakening one another to love.

Reconnecting in an Age of Separation

Two days after my life-threatening motorcycle accident some thirty-five years ago, I awoke in the ICU of Providence Santa Rosa Memorial Hospital with my crushed legs still intact and a body temperature of 105 degrees Fahrenheit. The intensive care staff managed to lower my temperature to 103 degrees, but it soon spiked up again. My doctors searched my body for the source of an infection or blood clot, but they were unsuccessful.

Meanwhile, my legs were being hoisted up, casted, and wrapped in bandages.

After what seemed like months, a young doctor came into my room, sat down beside me, and said cheerfully, "I have great news for you!"

"What is it?" I asked.

"We have thoroughly examined your body and found no signs of blood clots or infection," he replied. "We believe your high fever was just a reaction to the lengthy fifteen-hour surgery. You'll be walking out of here in a few days!"

I blinked at him in disbelief. "Did you see the lower half of this bed?" I asked. "Those are my casted legs down there."

The doctor glanced over, his face reddening. "Well, nowadays we all specialize in certain areas," he stammered. "Rehabilitation is outside my expertise."

That doctor lacked any sense that I was a whole human being. Once he found a medical explanation for my fever, his job was done. He failed to see me as anything more than a collection of symptoms written on a chart.

Decades later, while facing two life-threatening diagnoses simultaneously—nodular malignant melanoma and heart failure—I received the best medical care available from high-level medical experts at the University of California San Francisco School of Medicine. However, not one person of my very distinguished medical team ever asked how I was coping emotionally or offered support to my wife during these difficult times.

Despite miraculous advances in pain management and life extension, we have failed to establish comprehensive treatment plans for the human emotions at life's end. We build brilliant medical systems that too often see patients as bodies without feelings. Even with the best care, many of us face death alone in a hospital.

In this last chapter, I seek to explore an alternative: care that is centered on human connection and facilitated by psychedelics. This holistic approach to medicine sees each person as a whole human being. It helps us find meaning and transcend isolation, even—or perhaps especially—when in the process of dying. When life hangs in the balance, compassionate care matters most of all.

THE POWER OF COMPANIONSHIP

Modern life isolates us. Where we used to live in closely knit tribes, we now live anonymously among strangers—too often afraid of the small percentage of dangerous souls in our midst. The newspapers terrify us into avoiding public spaces—though the odds of harm remain small—and we become alienated by discomfort with our fellow beings. This discomfort builds walls where bonds once grew.

We live stacked in city skyscrapers, but we do not speak when in shared spaces. Elevators go up and down, containing people who stand in silence. Occupants have forgotten the art of casual conversation. We sit in theaters, movies, buses, trains, and airplanes without saying hello to the person next to us.

What was once unthinkable in tight-knit tribes now defines modern existence.

During the COVID pandemic, our isolation and alienation was dramatically intensified as people were mandated to shelter in place.

This worldwide pandemic demanded social distancing, and though our isolation may have temporarily protected our bodies, the friendly, social, and tribal animal in us despaired. Forced into our little rooms—be they single-room dwellings or mansion wings—we lost life's shared spaces, and moments of closeness with familiar others.

In ordinary times, we could still choose spaces of emotional warmth and welcome, but under lockdown we had only cold comfort—connecting with each other on pixelated screens—together but apart.

When the pandemic hit, those who were already living alone and without regular human interaction were hit the hardest.

Now that the pandemic is nearly over, we need to address the things that separate us, create relationships, and protect ourselves from alienation, hopelessness, and fear in the face of danger. We need structures that promote community, facilitate face-to-face connections, and raise morale. The things that matter, that have real value, are the connections we have with others, the people we know and care for rather than material possessions or financial accomplishments.

One of the recurring characters in this book has been my dear friend and neighbor, Charles Bush, who dedicated years of his life to serving the elderly as he himself was becoming an elder. Bush, one of the wisest philosophers I've encountered, is also the founder of prominent schools in Taos, New Mexico, and Mendocino, California. After a lifetime of teaching the young, Bush devoted his later years to understanding the experiences of those approaching death as the director of the Redwood Coast Seniors, a senior citizen center in Fort Bragg, California.

Seeking purpose after the 2008 recession, Bush found his way to the senior center by chance. He then spent twelve years with those nearing death, organizing community meals, transportation, and social events for hundreds of seniors every day.

"It was an incredible gift," he says. "After working with young people for so long, I got to work with the elderly and watched many pass away over the twelve years I worked there. About a quarter of the members died during that time."

Working at the senior center granted Bush an incredible sense of fulfillment. I remember him bussing dishes in the dining hall and greeting each resident by their name. His gift for cultivating community sprang from a lifetime of attending to human relationships and his willingness to show up fully for others. Bush helped transform the center into a place of connection and meaning during a time of life often marked more by isolation and confusion than companionship.

"My parents died when I was young," Bush tells me. "So by age sixty-five, I had never spent time with elderly people or known any elders well."

At first, Bush felt a distance between himself and the residents. It took several days of working in the dining hall for him to realize that "I was one of them—an elder, too— reaching the end of life."

Bush doesn't know how much time he has left. However, he tells me that he can feel in his bones that the final stretch has begun.

"Striking things happen as we age," he says, "First, we lose some of our mental and physical capacities—some of us faster than others. This loss of ability serves as an early warning that our bodies and minds will eventually wear out."

Like me, Bush is well into his eighties, although like me, he also shows little signs of slowing down.

While some find solace in religious beliefs about an afterlife, Bush discovered that most seniors at the center confronted death with uncertainty about the next step.

Housed in brilliant medical systems, he notes that, usually, people die in hospitals hooked up to machines, cut off from their community.

The process of dying, which can be shared collaboratively, often becomes a secret that is tucked away. We tend to avoid those who are dying and find their experience to be alien, sad, and depressing.

By avoiding the dying, or absenting ourselves from the moment of passing, or in the time leading up to it, we miss out on learning what they are experiencing.

Bush asked me, "How many people have you held, embraced or read to as they were dying, bit by bit?"

For the vast majority of us, myself included, the answer is few, if any.

Due to medical technology, death now occurs outside of the natural context of the home.

"It's no wonder that dying is such a mysterious and somewhat terrifying, somewhat confusing experience."

Which of us would choose to die in a hospital room?

Asked what it's like to die alone, Bush replied, "Well, by definition, we don't know. It might be horrifying, it might be wonderful. I don't know."

Bush envisions a better way to pass on. He suggested that, when we know the end is near, it's time for the whole family to come together. We should take time off work and gather at home to cook, share memories, and appreciate the time we have left.

In this model, dying would become a shared experience—not a secret. This, he says, could change who we are and change our culture as well.

He suggests that families might designate at least one family member who would receive time off from work for a loved one's passing—like maternity leave, but for the care of the soon-to-be-deceased instead of the recently-born. Bush notes. "Wouldn't it be marvelous if when somebody reaches that time of transition, that we release as many of the family and community as possible to spend as much time with them as possible?"

When the end is near, it's time for the whole family to come together. We are being counseled by a wise elder to take time off work and gather at home to cook, share memories, and appreciate—even celebrate—the time we have left. Transitioning leave can follow in the path of maternity leave.

When dying becomes an ordinary topic of conversation, it will be treated as naturally as being born. We come together for births and new life; we can also choose to come together for life's end before the funeral.

If we are to change the way we process dying in the way Bush suggests, the culture will need to change a bit first.

This is where psychedelic medicines come in. One of the most profound ways psychedelics can alleviate end-of-life distress is by fostering connections to people and nature, as well as enhancing meaning. This is not only true for the terminally ill patient who decides to undergo psychedelic-assisted psychotherapy, but also for anyone who comes in contact with a person during their "final stretch."

THE CALL FOR BETTER COMPANIONS

Offering psychedelics as treatment for end-of-life distress, brings with it the need for training and educating caregivers to bring the psychedelic frame of mind into their consciousness and the awareness of those they care for.

Caregivers spend the most tender moments with those nearing life's end. Their level of presence and compassion can stand large to patients and families alike. Psychedelic medicines offer caregivers a chance to cultivate qualities that serve families while offering emotional and physical comfort to the dying.

Andrew Penn, nurse practitioner and co-founder of the Organization of Psychedelic and Entheogenic Nurses, notes that nurses are natural candidates for administering end-of-life therapy with psychedelics. If 10 percent of nurses were versed in this care, as Andrew Penn suggests, we would have a huge workforce ready to serve those dying with empathy and grace.

"There are 3.8 million nurses in the United States—the largest healthcare profession," Penn tells me. "The pandemic underscored that a lot of nurses are burnt out and they're thinking about leaving the profession. I think a lot of them would stay if they could change what they're doing. Most nurses got into their profession because they wanted to help and heal people, and they still want that."

Andrew reports that the growing trends towards electronic health records and bureaucracy have discouraged many nurses and led to computer screen burnout. Many nurses despair of administrative tasks divorced from patient care. Psychedelic-assisted care lets the heart of nursing shine through.

Even 2 percent of the 3.8 million nurses would provide an extensive pool of nurses who already possess many of the fundamental skills required to be a psychedelic-assisted therapist, including being present with empathy, holding and controlling space with equanimity, and the ability to think and act with alacrity. Additionally, nurses are trained to provide care in the event of a physiological or psychological problem.

All of us crave human connection, yet the specialized systems and technology we have built around end-of-life care stand as obstacles to this connection. Nurses stand poised to remedy the isolation and dehumanization too common in modern systems of care.

Our systems must serve human needs for contact and compassion, not compete with them. There, psychedelic-trained nurses can lead the way.

Penn continues, "Nursing has a very important role in psychedelic work for a number of different reasons, some of which are obvious and practical. The psychedelic experience creates a long work day for the guide. However, being with a patient for six or eight hours is really not that unusual for a nurse. In nursing, a typical ICU shift is eight to twelve hours and you're with a patient who might be in an altered state of consciousness due to an illness. Being with a patient for a lengthy period of time and supporting them while they heal is a very familiar concept for nurses."

LETTING LOVED ONES HELP: A GIFT, NOT A BURDEN

Julie McFadden, the "TikTok Nurse," who moved from the ICU to hospice care, notes that it is often the family members of the dying who are most in need of therapy for their anxiety.

"Sometimes the family can be really difficult," she tells me. "People die how they lived, and families interact how they've always interacted."

Any serious illness, including end-of-life illnesses, requires family and caregivers to be mindful of their fears and apprehensions, as they can negatively impact the patient. The dying person looks to those around them, and fear in caregivers' eyes can be devastating. By projecting our own fears the person dying suffers. Psychedelic-assisted psychotherapy can help individuals come to terms with death as a natural part of the life cycle—an aspect that we all experience in life and can even celebrate at the end.

In the years before I began writing this book, I had little, if any, interest in thinking or talking about death. To me, death was as foreign a conversation topic as the moment before birth—both are part of the life cycle, and both are unknowable—case closed. These unknowns didn't seem worth my time. I asked myself why I should spend my precious lifetime talking about deathtime. For me death is simply a part of life that is inevitable and nothing to make a big thing about any more than all the other natural aspects of life.

One of my dearest friends, David Leonard Geisinger, Ph.D., had a fascination with death. He enjoyed talking and reading about it. His talk about death seemed gloomy to me. Until we change our cultural attitudes, death will remain a gloomy topic. David, past eighty, was on vacation with his wife, Lonnie Barbach, when he experienced a major stroke, which quickly led to his passing. After all his years of interest in death he managed a great way to go. No suffering and no pain. I keep a vibrant photo of him close and unabashedly live as though he is still in Mill Valley making dinner for Lonnie.

Another dear friend, Dr. James Guinan of Maumee, Ohio, died eighteen years ago at sixty-five. He walked into the shower, lost consciousness, and never regained it. He died clean but much too young. Upon getting word I immediately flew to Ohio in time to watch him being taken from the hospital room in a zipped up body bag. I maintain a relationship with Jim through his cowboy boots that he left with me. From time to time I speak to all of my friends who have passed. I know them enough that I make educated guesses as to their responses to my words. While of course I know this dialogue is make believe I find it enjoyable and comforting.

When my dad was in his mid-eighties, one morning, while visiting, I found him sitting on his bed crying. This was unusual for a military colonel and surgeon. In response to my query, he said sorrowfully, "I've outlived all my friends." After my wife and I had been together for ten years, we made a list of those we both knew who had passed. We quit the list last year when the list of those we knew who had died passed thirty. Now at eighty-five, so many of my own friends have transitioned. In addition, many of my most trusted business associates have retired or passed on. I deal with the loss by keeping some alive in my consciousness and delighting in the opportunity to meet new people in vivo. Recently, I have had the amazing good fortune of making friends with many people who could be my grandchildren. Luckily for me they are not ageists.

You may recall that since starting to write this book I have developed an interest in planning my own "grateful death," a going away party which I will be alive to attend. Within seventy-two hours of the end of the party I will transition to nothing, or something, as yet indescribable. I will call it my "going away party" but a gold watch or green bananas won't be necessary.

The idea of being able to choose when and where to transition is quite appealing to me. Just imagine all the interesting places and costumes one could choose for the occasion. I now envision a future where transitioning becomes a fun event.

Siobhan Greene, head of the Hospice Giving Foundation, credits me for my bravery in being willing to end my life with a lethal dose of something. However, she points out that many cannot do this for spiritual or practical reasons.

Furthermore, she suggests I reframe my view that needing care at the end of life would necessarily burden my loved ones. She argues that for many, providing care to someone who is dying can be a profound and meaningful experience.

"I would love for people to think of it more as not necessarily a burden," she tells me. "But an act of love to let somebody who has been so close and near and dear to you—somebody you love—care for you during your final days."

Although caring for dependent newborns is universally acknowledged as an act of love, we view dependence in old age as a burden, and wrongfully so. Viewing caring for those passing as a burden prevents the dying from accepting help from their families.

As for those who end up in the hospital or hospice under professional care, we might take comfort from Andrew Penn's comments that the nursing profession embraces the human component of their job as a refreshing break from the monotony of paperwork and bureaucracy.

Death Can Wait

I will come to death; it will not come to me. I will die when I want to die. If I sound arrogant, it is because death is arrogant. How dare death take my life? Let us focus on life and how we make meaning of our existence. Death can wait!

If any of you feel you must die right here and now, that is your choice. I trust the rest of you will join me in saying, death can wait . . . at least until we get home tonight.

I shall not allow my death to inconvenience my family and friends, and so I shall choose the time and place of my death. I am definitely choosing to remain alive right now. Death can wait. I wish we all believed we are going to live as long as we choose.

Let's look at what we gain and lose by believing we live as long as we choose. By living with the belief that we live as long as we choose, we live free of the fear of death lurking. By believing that death chooses us, we live with the sword of Damocles always hovering over our necks. When will the moment come? How much time do I have left?

Choosing the time and place of one's death will become the new normal. There will be great, colorful celebrations called goodbye parties that the soon dying will themselves attend rather than morbid, dressed-in-black funerals in which the celebrant participates while dead in a box. Which would you rather do?

Join me in making death a choice and departing with a celebration of life!

THERE'S MORE THAN MATERIALISM

We live in a world craving connection yet governed by materialism, each year losing ground in longevity and health. Anthony Bossis warns:

Within this field, I hope we don't lose sight of the importance of consciousness.

What is consciousness? Where is consciousness?

Why are we here?

We humans seem to have the capacity to be connected with some incredible insights.

Why would that be? To what end?

Why is the human design of consciousness so structured that we have the connection to experiences that provide people insights about death itself, and about why we're here?

Bossis urges finding "ways to house these numinous experiences" respecting their history and role in answering questions of consciousness and "why we're here." A premise of material gain bringing happiness "didn't come out to be true."

Despite advancing medically, America has recently seen a decline in life expectancy.

"There's something more than materialism," Bossis notes.

Psilocybin and other psychedelics have the potential to remind us of that something.

We live in an age of medical miracles yet often die alone, starved for connection and meaning. Though we may wish to avoid it, death awaits us all; what matters most is how we face that end—whether with acceptance, knowledge, and togetherness or anxiety, confusion, and distress—our fears hidden from our closest friends and family. The time for openness about our hopes for dying is now, before capacity or opportunity leave us wanting.

Whatever your age or health status, I ask you to imagine facing your own life's end: Do you wish to meet that moment alone or surrounded by familiar faces, hands held in moments of closeness too easily missed? For all we've gained in mobility and machines, we lost an art of dying suffused in human bonds within community. We built grand visions of global connection yet remain strangers in our own lives, disconnected from the immediate experience of death.

Psychedelic medicines may help reclaim the art of dying well while celebrating life. Psychedelics make the luminous accessible, help navigate space beyond small selves where human kinship feels most real. When our defenses fall, in loving-kindness we find a haven. Psychedelic care allows the dying to depart this life as all lives deserve to close—with dignity and surrounded by intimate others lighting the way ahead.

I want to close this chapter with a question from Charles Bush that is prominent on my inner TV screen.

"When you're dying, who do you want to have there?" Bush asked. His answer was even more memorable than his question.

You want those who are absolutely sure that consciousness is expansive, who absolutely dwell in loving kindness, and who have no problem with complete intimacy with you. Whether that means cleaning up after you while you're dying or feeding you carefully with fingers or a spoon, or just being there in complete silence or letting you scream in terror and holding onto you while also meeting you with complete peace and transparency.

Although some rare human beings come by these gifts of abundant generosity naturally, many of us need skill training to embody this kind of expansive consciousness.

The important thing, if we die together, is that at least one or two of us remain to hold hands and go, 'Let's leave together for a little while. You relax, I'll go out, we'll go together.'

And we would go to that holy place—that luminous place— where loving-kindness is not something you do. It's who and what you are, where the idea of different types of consciousness and areas of consciousness is as ordinary as anything could be, and there's no defense against intimacy.

Bush's wisdom reminds us that we must create room for expanded consciousness and support each other until the end of life and maybe even thereafter. By embracing the insights that psychedelics can provide, we gain access to wisdom that is as vast as the universe. This wisdom can help us move beyond our limited sense of self and connect with others in moments of intimacy that we might otherwise miss. In these moments of loving-kindness, we can let go of our defenses and find relief. Through this togetherness, life opens up and comes to a beautiful close, just as it began.

We can die gracefully.

EPILOGUE
The Way Forward

In my lifetime, I have witnessed a catastrophic policy failure unfold in slow motion: It is a war against people of color and alternate lifestyle people, the so-called "War on Drugs." As a psychologist, I have seen firsthand the damage wrought by this misguided campaign. It began in the 1930s when Harry Anslinger, the first commissioner of the Federal Bureau of Narcotics, effectively weaponized drug laws to target minorities and push a racist agenda. As chief drug warrior, Anslinger spread wild stories. He peddled in racist innuendo, saying that African Americans were giving cocaine to white women to have sex with them, and Hispanics who used marijuana became wild, uncontrollable rapists. He went on a campaign that eventually pushed other countries into making various substances illegal, creating the architecture for a global War on Drugs.

Prior to this War on Drugs, we didn't have mass epidemics of addiction; we had medical doctors taking care of people with chemical dependence.

We have spent billions of dollars and destroyed countless lives enforcing laws against psychedelic drugs that are less harmful and addictive than legal substances like alcohol or tobacco.

We learned from alcohol prohibition that people will continue to use substances whether they are legal or not. When prohibition ended, people didn't drink more or less than before, the government just gained taxation and control. Today, the situation with drug prohibition is very similar to alcohol prohibition, where outlawing a substance only spawns illegal activity and gives rise to criminal empires. As a result of this failed government policy, we have narco-cartels with so much money and power that they have taken over entire governments and compete with other governments for control of territory.

Furthermore, Anslinger turned police forces around the nations from peace officers into violent enforcers of unjust laws. More often than not, they targeted minorities and vulnerable communities.

As police lieutenant Sarko Gergerian told me, "Policing those laws has morally injured a lot of our first responders."

Ironically, we are now treating the very same police officers who have been psychologically injured with PTSD in the line of duty with the same substances that they have been tasked with policing for the past eighty plus years.

As the legal landscape around psychedelics shifts, we will need to be prepared with the proper containers and frameworks for safe and effective treatment. It is important that we give some thought and attention to easing this transition—the birth of a new field of medicine—coming out of the renaissance in research that has been under way these past ten years.

THE CHANGING LEGAL LANDSCAPE OF PSYCHEDELICS

Of all the psychedelics, MDMA seems most likely to have its legal status changed first. Thanks to the successful completion of Phase 2 clinical trials and the promising results of Phase 3 trials now under way, MDMA may be approved by the FDA for the treatment of PTSD before this book is published in late 2024.

Rescheduling MDMA from DEA's Schedule 1 of controlled substances to Schedule 2 or Schedule 3 will allow it to be legally administered by physicians and therapists.

Some proponents hype the potential benefits of rescheduling, imagining it will make MDMA available for recreational use. But as Andrew Penn cautions, "FDA approval doesn't make MDMA legal for general use, and that may come as a disappointment to some people."

MDMA would remain a controlled substance, available only through specialized clinics and trained professionals. Penn explains to me that rescheduling MDMA will be like the regulations around surgical anesthetics or buprenorphine for opioid addiction: legal for medical purposes, but administered in a specific setting.

The regulatory controls would be determined as part of a Risk Evaluation and Mitigation Strategy (REMS) that governs how the drug can be prescribed and used. For example, patients using Spravato, a ketamine-based nasal spray, must undergo two hours of observation following treatment. We can expect similar precautions for MDMA.

Rescheduling is a victory but is not outright legalization. MDMA will remain tightly regulated, though this framework can also reassure patients and professionals of its safe administration.

The hype around legalization often overlooks these important nuances.

With rescheduling, the medical establishment and pharmaceutical companies stand to gain a degree of control over psychedelics.

Some see this as threatening to limit access, creating a "priesthood" that guards these medicines. However, regulation also helps ensure quality of the medicine and of care. As UCLA researcher Grob argues, therapists require proper training and licensing to responsibly handle psychedelic treatments.

"However, my views tend to veer a bit towards the conservative," Grob tells me.

"The advantage of a trained health professional, a trained mental health professional, is that we have seen a lot of psychopathology, and if we're paying attention, we get good at identifying it when we see it," he says.

Licensing also deters reckless behavior by giving therapists "skin in the game." If rules are broken, they stand to lose their license. That's not the case with many underground therapists, who may stand to be penalized criminally or civilly, but who may have little to lose if they lack physical assets.

To those who worry that the medical profession may be trying to create a cartel or monopoly on prescription psychedelics, psilocybin mushrooms present an interesting case study. As organic as cannabis, psilocybin can be easily grown and cannot be regulated like many synthetic drugs.

The medical establishment may gain some control over access to synthesized psilocybin compounds, but natural psilocybin will remain hard to regulate. Patients may choose to undergo treatment at the hands of a licensed professional, using pharmaceutical-grade mushrooms or synthetic alternatives, or they may find an underground guide and cultivate their own supply.

LEGALIZATION VS. DECRIMINALIZATION— REGULATING QUALITY OF CARE

We are in a time of transition with psychedelics. Psychedelic substances remain illegal under federal law, though some cities and states have decriminalized some of them. Decriminalization means jurisdictions agree not to prosecute illegal acts, but there are currently no guidelines in place on who can administer these substances. By contrast, legalization supersedes decriminalization—allowing regulation to ensure safety as well as prosecution of those who violate these regulations.

I believe that individuals have a right to ingest anything they choose—as long as they are not harming others. Rat poison and heroin, for example, are dangerous but individuals have the right to use them. The law exists to stop harm to others—not to regulate personal intoxication or altered states of mind.

Legalization would allow specific guidelines as to who can administer psychedelics. Driving a car is legal but requires a license to ensure safety. Similarly, legalizing psilocybin could allow it to be prescribed by those with a license.

Decriminalization alone creates a risk of unsafe practices, but an overly restrictive medicalized model also risks limiting access to patients who need it most.

The medical establishment could have incentives to limit competition. Katherine MacLean expresses suspicion about the medical community's sudden interest in psychedelics.

"My vision for people and the planet is that they discover the safest and kindest way to practice releasing their fears," she says, "Whether that involves psychedelics or something else."

We also must expand access to more affordable options, such as group therapy and new categories of licensed professionals, for example "psychedelic coaches," who may not have an official license but who are trained in helping people navigate their fears and other difficulties that may arise during a psychedelic experience.

Legal and decriminalization models can coexist, for example, doctors prescribing psilocybin, but nondoctors also administering without prosecution. Based on trends in Oregon, Colorado, and California, we may see much of the nation decriminalize psychedelics before legalizing them. Some seventeen U.S. cities have already decriminalized psilocybin.

NEW MODELS FOR TRANSFORMATION

Once it's legal to do so, MAPS plans to train 25,000 psychedelic guides. Having guides—certified or underground—requires less training than doctors, lowering the costs of treatment, and new categories of licensed professionals can meet demand where psychiatrists are scarce. But we must avoid the hype of psychedelics being a panacea and instead walk this new path with care.

Writer Don Lattin cautions, "Psychedelics didn't save the world in the 1960s and won't in the 2020s."

Yet Lattin still sees a world ripe with potential. He recommends watching how religious groups incorporate psychedelics into their community and rituals. "I've been going to various churches that are forming or coming above ground now. I think that's an interesting area to watch," Lattin says.

Psychedelics have long been intertwined with spiritual seeking, though often underground. Hunt Priest, founder of Ligare, represents a growing openness around psychedelics in religious contexts. He believes that psychedelics, which catalyzed his vision, will resonate even with Christians wary of "drugs." Through education and retreats, he aspires to expand access to entheogens as aids for spiritual growth.

Priest doesn't envision psychedelics replacing the usual Sunday-morning sacraments like some more radical psychedelic preachers do. Instead, he envisions retreats where Christians can encounter the divine and integrate psychedelic lessons into daily life. He pictures five-day retreats incorporating Bible study, prayer, meditation, and sacraments from the Christian tradition and psychedelics.

"On day three, there might be a facilitated psilocybin experience," he says. "Psilocybin lends itself well to a retreat context, as its effects only last about six hours."

The final retreat days would involve integrating insights from the psychedelic experience into everyday life. Like the Old Testament prophets returning from divine encounters with God, participants at psychedelic retreats will discern how to apply revelations about themselves, God, and others.

"You try to figure out how to live your life knowing what you've experienced," Priest says. Just as Moses descended from Mount Sinai transformed, retreat goers come down the mountain and back into the world equipped with lessons for the journey ahead.

Priest aspires to make such psychedelic communion available to all who seek it, not just an elite few. "This is not about profit, ownership or control," he says. "It's about bringing healing to whoever wants it."

Through education and leading by example, Priest hopes to see more mainstream religious institutions adopt this path of risk and revelation.

Similarly, Thomas Roberts, the first professor to teach a for-credit university course on psychedelic studies, which he did at Northern Illinois University, is trying to interest a men's group at his church in the idea.

Roberts also believes that seniors in particular would benefit from education on responsible use of psychedelics. "I've taught several psychedelic courses in our local senior center groups that were very well attended," he says. "Seniors make great students. They attend because they want to learn."

By educating new professional groups to supplement the work of mental health professionals, we establish an integrated network to meet demand for psychedelic medicine responsibly.

ON OLD AGE: REFLECTIONS OF
A PSYCHEDELIC ELDER

The real antidote to end-of-life distress is not just acceptance of death, but living life to the fullest, at any age. The Roman philosopher Cicero, in his essay "On Old Age," argued that the second half of life, however long it may be, offers abundant opportunities for meaning and fulfillment.

For Cicero, old age need not be a time of decline, but an apex of wisdom and vitality.

"My house is not just full, but overflowing with callers," he writes. Even in one's later years, satisfying connections and contributions remain possible.

I also prescribe an active life, grounded in friends and family, exercise, and purposeful pastimes. Cicero urged elders to maintain vigor and cheerfulness, to keep learning, and cultivate friendships across generations. Above all, he advised continued participation in public affairs.

"Old age," wrote Cicero, "will only be respected if it fights for itself, maintains its rights, submits to no one, and rules over its domain until its last breath."

Psychedelics, when used wisely, can help seniors maintain the sort of dynamic engagement Cicero described. By overcoming excessive anxiety and attachment, psychedelics allow people to live each day to the fullest, all the way up to the end.

My own vitality today, at eighty-five years old, stems partly from psychedelic sessions, which have repeatedly shown me that consciousness exists beyond the body. This attitude liberates me to live fully, seizing each day as the gift it is.

Yet, again: psychedelics are not magic bullets. Psychedelic experiences provide glimpses of deeper realities, but we must do the work to actualize them. Lasting changes in how we engage life require rigorous integration after the psychedelic journey. We cannot simply trip our way to fulfillment.

Cicero's prescription applies here: continued learning, service, exercise, moderation, and social bonds fortify us to age with strength and purpose. So, while overcoming the fear of death is crucial, the key to aging well is continuing to live fully and deeply.

My hope is for these psychedelic medicines to become increasingly available; with proper containers and guidance, they can, and will, unlock suppressed wisdom and vitality at any age.

Nevertheless, this psychedelic renaissance requires us to walk carefully. As laws and attitudes shift, we must balance safety and access, guarding against both draconian restrictions and reckless freedoms. Communities, professionals, and lawmakers all have their roles to play.

There will likely be setbacks amid progress. Psychedelic plants and chemicals are tools that can profoundly heal but they may also be deeply disruptive when used improperly. It is our task to advance judiciously and avoid overhyping benefits.

Still, the suffering that psychedelics address is so widespread and devastating that their continued suppression cannot be justified. Epidemiologists inform me that 30 to 40 percent of the United States suffers from anxiety and depression. I am hopeful that within my lifetime appropriate legal regulation will enable trained professionals to prescribe these medicines, which address this emotional dis-ease.

As my friend, police lieutenant Sarko Gergerian says, "What an amazing country we live in where we have the freedoms and rights that are sacred and enshrined in our Constitution and in our founding documents. This is one of the most amazing countries on Earth in my opinion, and it deserves reverence and care, and we need to keep working to make it better, all of us."

And as laws evolve, each of us must care for our minds, bodies, and relationships with deliberation. Rather than accepting mortality when it arrives, we are called to vigorously engage each precious day we're granted. May our policies, communities, and day-to-day choices all increasingly reflect and honor this sacred vision of each of us having a life well spent.

In concluding this chapter and book, I return to hope—the hope of ending repressive policies causing vast and unnecessary suffering, and hope of allowing access to the effective healing that psychedelic medicines offer. The hope that we can build a society that honors the sacredness of each life.

And last, but always first, I remain hopeful that we will create an alternative to our capitalistic financial system, which intrinsically favors the very few and does devastating damage to the many.

Afterword

There are times in our lives when each of us will be called upon to decide whether, or not, to ingest into our being a foreign substance, called medicine, for the purpose of enhancing our psychophysical well-being. We take the medicine in hope of relief or cure. We each make the decision about taking the medicine in our own way. Some of us rely on experts often called doctors. Some of us rely on folklore or what others who have ingested the medicine report. Some of us are facile with the internet and research the medicine to the best of our ability. Some do all of the above and even more. We each make a bet on whether or not to ingest the medicine related to our perceived relationship of reward and risk. A certain percentage of the population are so easily influenced by the opinion of "leaders" that national admissions to ER rooms for poison went up significantly after Donald Trump announced to America that disinfectants cure COVID.

The vast majority simply follow their doctor's prescription and take whatever it is the doctor tells them to take.

And now cometh a new medicine called psychedelic that effects body, mind, and spirit and that brings with it the highest hopes along with a controversial reputation.

The very notion of taking a psychedelic medicine will be accepted quite differently depending on what the culture was promoting during one's formative years. For those who bought into the media hype of people on psychedelics jumping out of buildings, taking a psychedelic while fearful of dying would be like jumping out of a plane as a way of getting over fear of heights. (I did once treat a person with a flying phobia on a commercial airline flight.)

On the other end of the cultural continuum are those tens of millions who have experimented with psychedelics and recognize their potential health-enhancing value.

And then there is the vast majority of our citizenry, the great middle, who are honestly uncertain.

For those who, for a myriad of reasons, did not succumb to the fearmongering and instead look to be guided by science as referenced throughout this book, and for those simply brave at heart, psychedelic medicines at the end of life, especially for those who have dis-ease about dying, are an option with great merit.

References

Anderson, Brian T., Alicia Danforth, Robert Daroff, et al. 2020. "Psilocybin-Assisted Group Therapy for Demoralized Older Long-Term AIDS Survivor Men: An Open-Label Safety and Feasibility Pilot Study." *EClinical Medicine* 24, no. 27 (September): 100538.

Babyak, Michael, James Blumenthal, Steve Herman, Parinda Khatri, Murali Doraiswamy, Kathleen Moore, Teri Baldewicz, Ranga Krishnan, and Edward Craighead. 2000. "Exercise Treatment for Major Depression: Maintenance of Therapeutic Benefit at 10 Months." *Psychosomatic Medicine* 62, no. 5 (September–October): 633–38.

Baribeau, Renee. 2018. *Winds of Spirit: Ancient Wisdom Tools for Navigating Relationships, Health, and the Divine.* Carlsbad, CA: Hay House.

Baum, Dan. 2016. "Legalize It All." *Harper's Magazine*, April.

Buchanan, John H., 2022. *Processing Reality: Finding Meaning in Death, Psychedelics, and Sobriety.* Eugene, OR: Cascade Books.

Byock, Ira. 2012. *The Best Care Possible: A Physician's Quest to Transform Care Through the End of Life.* New York: Avery.

Byock, Ira. 2018. "Taking Psychedelics Seriously." *Journal of Palliative Medicine* 21 no. 4 (April 1): 417–21.

Carhart-Harris, R. L., M. Bolstridge, C. M. J. Day, et al. 2018. "Psilocybin with Psychological Support for Treatment-Resistant Depression: Six-Month Follow-Up." *Psychopharmacology* 235, no. 2: 399–408.

CDC. 2022. "Overweight and Obesity: Adult Obesity Facts." CDC website. Accessed March 9, 2023.

Compass Pathways. 2021. "Open-Label Study of COMP360 Psilocybin Therapy for Depression in Cancer Patients Demonstrates Feasibility of Simultaneous Psilocybin Administration in Small Groups." Yahoo Finance website, October 20.

Daws, Richard E., Christopher Timmermann, Bruna Giribaldi, James D. Sexton, Matthew B. Wall, David Erritzoe, Leor Roseman, David Nutt, and Robin Carhart-Harris. 2022. "Increased Global Integration in the Brain after Psilocybin Therapy for Depression." *Nature Medicine* 28: 844–51.

de Wit, Harriet. 2006. "Towards a Science of Spiritual Experience." *Psychopharmacology* 187, 267.

Dickler, Jessica. 2023. "62% of Americans Are Still Living Paycheck to Paycheck, Making It 'The Main Financial Lifestyle,' Report Finds." CNBC website (October 31).

Garcia-Romeu, Albert, Alan K. Davis, Fire Erowid, Earth Erowid, Roland R. Griffiths, Matthew W. Johnson. 2019. "Cessation and Reduction in Alcohol Consumption and Misuse after Psychedelic Use." *Journal of Psychopharmacology* 33, no. 2 (September): 1088–1101.

Griffiths, Roland R., William A. Richards, Una McCann, and Robert Jesse. 2006. "Psilocybin Can Occasion Mystical-Type Experiences Having Substantial and Sustained Personal Meaning and Spiritual Significance." *Psychopharmacology (Berl)* 187, no. 3 (August): 268–83; discussion 284–92.

Griffiths, Roland, Matthew W. Johnson, Michael A Carducci, Annie Umbricht, William A. Richards, Brian D. Richards, Mary P. Cosimano, Margaret A. Klinedinst. 2016. "Psilocybin Produces Substantial and Sustained Decreases in Depression and Anxiety in Patients with Life-Threatening Cancer: A Randomized Double-Blind Trial." *Journal of Psychopharmacology.* 30, no. 12 (December): 1181–97.

Grob, C. S., A. L. Danforth, G. S. Chopra, M. Hagerty, C. R. McKay, A. L. Halberstadt, G. R. Greer. 2011. "Pilot Study of Psilocybin Treatment for Anxiety in Patients with Advanced-Stage Cancer." *Archives of General Psychiatry* 68, no. 1 (January): 71–78.

Heinlein, Robert. 1987. *Stranger in a Strange Land.* New York: Ace.

Hood Jr, Ralph W., and Ronald J. Morris. 1983. "Toward a Theory of Death Transcendence." *Journal for the Scientific Study of Religion* 22, no. 4: 353–65.

Huxley, Laura. 1963. Letter to Julian Huxley (December 8). Available on the Library of Consciousness website under "A Beautiful Death."

Marinacci, Michael. 2023. *Psychedelic Cults and Outlaw Churches.* Rochester, VT: Park Street Press.

Lattin, Don. 2010. *The Harvard Psychedelic Club: How Timothy Leary, Ram Dass, Huston Smith, and Andrew Weil Killed the Fifties and Ushered in a New Age for America*. HarperOne.

Lattin, Don. 2023. *God on Psychedelics: Tripping Across the Rubble of Old-Time Religion*. Berkeley, CA: Apocryphile Press.

Khamsehzadeh, Jahan. 2022. *The Psilocybin Connection: Psychedelics, The Transformation of Consciousness, and Evolution on the Planet*. Berkeley, CA: North Atlantic Books.

MacLean, Katherine. 2023. *Midnight Water*. Brattleboro, VT: Green Writers Press.

MacLean, Katherine A., Matthew W. Johnson, and Roland R. Griffiths. 2011. "Mystical Experiences Occasioned by the Hallucinogen Psilocybin Lead to Increases in the Personality Domain of Openness." *Journal of Psychopharmacology* 25, no. 11: 1453–61.

MacLean, Katherine A., Jeannie-Marie S Leoutsakos, and R. Griffiths. 2012. "Factor Analysis of the Mystical Experience Questionnaire: A Study of Experiences Occasioned by the Hallucinogen Psilocybin." *Journal for the Scientific Study of Religion* 4:721–37.

Miller, Richard Louis. 2017. *Psychedelic Medicine: The Healing Power of LSD, MDMA, Psilocybin and Ayahuasca*. Rochester, VT: Park Street Press.

Miller, Richard Louis. 2022. *Psychedelic Wisdom: The Astonishing Rewards of Mind-Altering Substances*. Rochester, VT: Park Street Press.

Mitchell, Jennifer M., G. Ot'alora, B. van der Kolk, et al. 2023. "MDMA-Assisted Therapy for Moderate to Severe PTSD: A Randomized, Placebo-Controlled Phase 3 Trial." *Nature Medicine* 29: 2473–80.

Moreno, Francisco A, Christopher B. Wiegand, E. Keolani Taitano, and Pedro L. Delgado. 2006. "Safety, Tolerability, and Efficacy of Psilocybin in 9 Patients with Obsessive-Compulsive Disorder." *Journal of Clinical Psychiatry* 67, no. 11 (November): 1735–40.

Nichols, D. E. 2006. "Commentaries and Editorial on Article By Griffiths et al. 'Psilocybin Can Occasion Mystical-Type Experiences Having Substantial and Sustained Personal Meaning and Spiritual Significance.'" *Psychopharmacology* 187, no. 3: 268–69.

Pollan, Michael. 2018. *How to Change Your Mind*. New York: Penguin.

Pollan, Michael. 2022. *How to Change Your Mind*. Netflix miniseries.

Psychedelic Support Network. 2023. "How To Join a Psychedelic Clinical Trial." Psychedelic Support Network website. Accessed February 7, 2023.

Raison, Charles L., Gerard Sanacora, Joshua Woolley, et al. 2023. "Single-Dose Psilocybin Treatment for Major Depressive Disorder: A Randomized Clinical Trial." *JAMA* 330, no. 9: 843–53.

Roberts, Thomas. 2019. *MindApps: Multistate Theory and Tools for Mind Design*. Rochester, VT: Park Street Press.

Ross, Stephen, Anthony Bossis , Jeffrey Guss, et al. 2016. "Rapid and Sustained Symptom Reduction Following Psilocybin Treatment for Anxiety and Depression in Patients with Life-Threatening Cancer: A Randomized Controlled Trial." *Journal of Psychopharmacology* 30, no. 12: 1165–80.

Sjöstedt-Hughes, Peter. 2015. *Noumenautics: Metaphysics—Meta-ethics—Psychedelics*. UK: Psychedelic Press.

Sjöstedt-Hughes, Peter. 2021. *Modes of Sentience: Psychedelics, Metaphysics, Panpsychism*. UK: Psychedelic Press.

Sjöstedt-Hughes Peter. 2023. "On the Need for Metaphysics in Psychedelic Therapy and Research." *Frontiers in Psychology* 14 (March 30): 1128589.

Woolley, Joshua. 2021. "Psilocybin Therapy for Depression and Anxiety in Parkinson's Disease: A Pilot Study." ID NCT04932434. UCSF Clinical Trials website. Accessed March 9, 2024.

Index